QM Medical Libraries

24 1017521 6

D0550335

Weight Matters for Children

A complete guide to weight, eating and fitness

Rachel Pryke
General Practitioner
Member, Worcestershire Obesity Reduction and Prevention Strategy Group

Forewords by

Joe Harvey
Director
Health Education Trust

and

Annabel Karmel

WITHDRAWN
FROM STOCK
QMUL LIBRARY

Radcliffe Publishing
Oxford • Seattle

Radcliffe Publishing Ltd
18 Marcham Road
Abingdon
Oxon OX14 1AA
United Kingdom

www.radcliffe-oxford.com
Electronic catalogue and worldwide online ordering facility.

_____

© 2006 Rachel Pryke

All rights reserved. No part of this publication may be reproduced, stored in a retrieval system or transmitted, in any form or by any means, electronic, mechanical, photocopying, recording or otherwise without the prior permission of the copyright owner.

British Library Cataloguing in Publication Data

A catalogue record for this book is available from the British Library.

ISBN 1 85775 771 8

BARTS & THE LONDON QMSMD	
CLASS MARK	WS130 PRY
CIRC TYPE	ORD
SUPPLIER	CISL £14.95 13|2|06
READING LIST	
OLD ED CHECK	

Typeset by Anne Joshua & Associates, Oxford
Printed and bound by TJ International Ltd, Padstow, Cornwall

Contents

Foreword

Understanding how a process works is vital when planning successful changes. In this book, Rachel Pryke sets out a framework to enable parents and carers to positively manage the increasingly challenging task of keeping a child's lifestyle healthy.

Anyone doubting the value of such a book has only to look around at the now familiar sight of overweight adults and children in our society or witness the anxiety provoked by a child that will not eat at all. Look at the supermarket shelves lined with processed and pre-prepared products; watch parents of young children running the gauntlet of supermarket checkouts lined with sweets. Try spending a Saturday morning watching children's television on the commercial channels to witness that the level of advertising of a product is in inverse ratio to its nutritional value. National and multinational food producers do not apply the enormous marketing pressure to purchase their 'added value' goods for the benefit of our children but to give best return to their shareholders.

Even though recent attention has quite properly focused on improving the quality of foods in our schools, it must be remembered that the most important influences in the development of a child's dietary habits are in the home. For the first four years home influences are paramount, and even for the 40% of youngsters who go on to have school lunches, this is only one meal in the day for five days a week and for only 40 weeks of the year.

Although we would all like to build good habits from the start, putting ideals into practice is not always straightforward. Parenting is tough enough without having to cope with the blandishments of the food industry, the often well-intended but sometimes conflicting input from grandparents, the tempting nature of ready meals for those exhausted moments and the worries that well-publicised food scares bring.

This book is a very practical, thoughtful and parent/carer friendly resource aimed at supporting both the planning of family meals and the troubleshooting that will inevitably be needed from time to time. Crucially it makes clear the vital importance of balancing the equation between intake of food and energy output from physical activity.

Within, a wealth of common sense sits alongside sound child psychology which underpins the advice throughout the text. The knowledge that Rachel brings to the book as a mother and an experienced family doctor adds real value which informs and reassures. I remember clearly some of the battles, most won but some lost, for the hearts and minds of my own children in encouraging them to eat well and get real pleasure from food – this book would have been invaluable to me then and certainly will be to its readers now.

Joe Harvey
Director, Health Education Trust
October 2005

Foreword

What you feed your child today will determine his future tomorrow. In the first year babies happily enjoy eating foods without added sugar or salt. Unfortunately as they grow older their diet deteriorates rapidly and over the last decade we have seen the emergence of a new food category, 'children's food'. More often than not this represents some of the worst quality foods on offer, high in saturated fat, sugar or salt. Whether it's a sugary refined breakfast cereal, a lunchbox snack which contains almost as much salt as a young child should eat in an entire day or a juice drink which contains just 6% juice and 94% sugar and water, children will soon develop a taste for fried, salty or excessively sweet foods, and fresh produce may seem bland and boring in comparison.

More and more children and adolescents are now overweight or obese. One in five children in the UK is now overweight. Fast food and poor quality ready-to-eat meals are becoming a regular part of the average diet. These processed foods account for 75% of the saturated fat and salt that children consume. If we want our children to grow up healthy and strong we need to include more fresh foods in their diets.

Cooking healthy meals doesn't mean you have to spend hours in the kitchen. There are lots of ways to get children to improve their diet – for example, whilst fruit in a fruit bowl is seldom eaten, cut it into bite size pieces and thread it onto a skewer or straw and it becomes a treat. After school kids are generally starving but the only food on offer tends to be a bag of crisps or a chocolate biscuit – take a few minutes to prepare some healthy snacks and leave them on a low shelf in the fridge where your child can go and help himself. Make 'healthy junk food' – home made burgers, pizzas, chicken nuggets – from good quality ingredients. For fussy children you may need to resort to disguising and preparing a hidden vegetable tomato sauce for pasta where six different vegetables are blended into the sauce, and what children can't see, they can't pick out . . .

We know that children who eat a healthy diet have improved levels of concentration and so perform better at school. We also know that children who are overweight have lower levels of self-esteem and are often unhappy. Rachel Pryke gives lots of good advice on how to improve your child's diet and set them up for a happy and healthy future.

Annabel Karmel
October 2005

Annabel has written 14 books on healthy food for babies and children including *Annabel Karmel's New Complete Baby and Toddler Meal Planner* (Ebury Press, 2004) and *Annabel Karmel's Favourite Family Recipes* (Ebury Press, 2005). She also has her own website, www.annabelkarmel.com.

Preface

This book is for everyone who would like to see healthy children enjoying great food and plenty of activity. A child's build counts towards far more than physical appearance alone: self-confidence and personal pride, fitness and susceptibility to illness will all stem from a child's diet. Eating and exercise habits that begin in childhood are likely to last for life and so getting the basics right is one of the best investments a child can have.

Weight Matters for Children provides the best and most up-to-date evidence on understanding children's choices and their motivation, plus a complete summary of childhood nutrition, from additives to vegetables. It ranges from putting a healthy diet into practice, binning barriers to exercise, tackling bullying and low self-esteem, right through to an A to Z of common conditions and illnesses that are related to diet or physical health. It uses the United Kingdom (UK) national food guide, *The Balance of Good Health*, to help family meals fit the bill and to bring a consistent message into the home, because this is the same easy nutritional system that is taught to children in UK schools.

Weight Matters for Children explains how families may slip into unhealthy habits – and how they can get back on track once more! From baby's first mouthful of milk, through the fussy years of toddlerdom and into the junior years of advertising and peer pressure, busy parents and choosy children can learn how to live healthily despite hectic or chaotic lives. By taking a look at how children make up their minds over daily decisions, including how parents weigh into that process, families can discover simple and achievable approaches that will help children to make healthy choices for themselves, regardless of whether parents are there to insist or not.

With so much confusing dietary advice and heavy advertising of unhealthy foods it can be hard to know where to go for reliable information. Inside, all the nutritional information is consistent with highly respected sources ranging from The British Heart Foundation, The Food Standards Agency, The Food Commission and the World Health Organization. It is also fully consistent with *Preventing Childhood Obesity* (BMA, June 2005).

As a parent who has spent years fretting over the eating habits of my own three boys, I have written the book with other parents in mind. But at the same time, I am also a doctor who has been treating families for 16 years and so I feel confident that health professionals will find the book a useful compilation of the best current nutritional advice – plus how to put it into practice! I hope it will be useful both for families and for health professionals to recommend when a reliable source of further information is required.

Rachel Pryke
October 2005

About the author

Rachel Pryke MBBS, MRCGP trained at King's College Hospital, London. She is now a GP in Worcestershire with particular interests in family medicine, women's health and weight management. She is a regular contributor to medical magazines and writes on a wide variety of topics.

In *Weight Matters for Children* she has combined the most up-to-date evidence and advice on childhood nutrition and child psychology with the practical knowledge that comes from being both a practising doctor and a parent.

Rachel comes from a medical and musical family and is married to a GP. They have three boys plus a naughty shoe-stealing dog called Tiffin.

Acknowledgements

I would like to thank the following people for their suggestions and encouragement. My biggest thanks go to Sally and Lyndon Simkin, whose guidance and enthusiasm has been constant and highly constructive. I am also indebted to Laurel Forster for her succinct and canny assessment of early drafts, which enabled me to move swiftly along the learning curve. It is a joy to have useful friends!

Further thanks for chapter reading and general support go to Marie-Claire Parsons, Anne Maloney, Julian Davey, Deborah Hugh, Sonia Oliver and Penny Dowley. Helen Mercer provided valuable nutritional input, thank you.

Thank you to Joe Harvey of the Health Education Trust for his help and support. My thanks also go to John Short for all his help in providing growth charts and to Tam Fry, of the Child Growth Foundation, for his generosity in allowing his material to be made available.

I am grateful to Tamar Karet for her input into the original concept. My warmest appreciation goes to Tom, Alistair, Abigail and children of RGS The Grange School, Worcester, for their lovely artwork as used on the cover.

I would have been lost without the constant support and encouragement from my family, and so my love and thanks go to them always.

Lastly, I am very grateful to Radcliffe Publishing, in particular to Gillian Nineham, for taking on such a novice.

To my beloved boys: Tom, Alistair, Bertie and, of course, David.

Section 1

Children and choice

The first three introductory chapters look at some of the basic principles of how children choose things for themselves and what motivates them to join in and take part. It outlines a healthy eating plan for all the family and describes how to check up on a child's growth. These principles and ideas are used throughout the book to show how small changes to current lifestyles can make a big difference to a child's health.

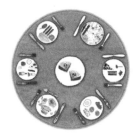

Chapter 1

Children, choices and *The Balance of Good Health*

Who is in charge of how children eat?

This question has many answers ranging from the government, the food industry, supermarket managers, corner shop assistants and even dinner ladies. As for parents and children themselves, how much control do they really have over meals and snacks when they are manipulated by supermarkets into buying whatever is on offer and when advertisements tell children what to like? This book shows how families can step in to take control over how they eat and put health and fitness successfully onto the family priority list.

It is a traditional view that in order for children to do what is good for them, they must be told what to do. In many circumstances this is true, and in some food settings this will work. Children do not automatically like things that are good for them and have to develop a taste for different foods but, as many parents will readily testify, telling a child to eat his greens is a thankless and often fruitless endeavour. Indeed, forcing disliked foods may simply harden the child's resolve to avoid what is being pushed altogether. This is the 'catch- 22' situation: how can children be persuaded to keep trying new things that take some getting used to and to eat less of the tasty foods that are not so good for them?

There are many avenues to help children make happy, healthy choices for themselves. Childhood is a time for experimenting with choice, when adults are around to guide the process. The more people understand how children make choices the greater the chance of helping them continue to make good choices when parents are not around.

Children learn about making choices from the following factors:

- copying parents and other role models
- the choice worked last time, i.e. they are choosing something familiar
- the choice might annoy parents, and that can be fun
- the choice was relevant to them, i.e. they sensed it was good for them
- they could not think of a good alternative, i.e. that's how the family do things
- the choice was easy, rather than an effort
- they had some control over the choice, even if that meant getting it wrong, i.e. it *was* a choice.

It is worrying that so many of today's children are making poor choices about how they eat. Despite having a wider choice of foods than ever before, children do not seem to be getting the balance right. Newspapers are full of headlines about the 'obesity epidemic' that is sweeping the western world. Even children who are of normal weight for their height may not be eating enough fresh produce to ensure good health, which may put them at higher risk of developing illnesses as they get older.

Whilst parents may have a reasonable idea as to what they would like their kids to eat, getting them to eat it is an entirely different matter. Happily there is plenty of good advice to follow with helpful healthy eating guidelines produced by many governments in different countries. This book uses United Kingdom (UK) nutritional guidelines and gives helpful ideas on how to fit these guidelines into daily family life.

Some examples are the Department of Health's 'Take Five' or 'Five-A-Day' campaign that encourages everyone to eat at least five portions of fruit and vegetables each day. Another is the Food Standards Agency's *The Balance of Good Health* food guide, which is used throughout this book and which is taught to children in schools as part of personal, social and health education. Because the book explores how children make up their minds and the things that influence choice, parents will discover not only which guidelines to follow but also how to make them work.

Start with establishing healthy basics

The key to a healthy diet is getting the balance right. Many eating surveys have shown that high-fat diets are strongly linked to becoming overweight. A high-fat diet tends to contain a small amount of fruit and vegetables whereas people eating lower-fat diets tend to eat far more fruit and vegetables. If families focus on eating more fruit and vegetables then the overall diet will become better balanced without having to fuss especially over the fat content. It is a case of getting the basics right so that other details will not be so significant.

Whilst this sounds simple, many parents struggle because their children are reluctant to choose plain healthy foods when there is a ready supply of tastier and more satisfying options. In order to help children choose healthily we need to understand what sways their choices. This has been extensively studied by the Department of Nutrition at Pennsylvania State University in the United States, and its approaches have now been incorporated into the most up-to-date guidelines on healthy eating for children. In particular it has shed light on how children make choices and why they might like something or not. A fundamental finding – which might appear almost too obvious to mention – is that *children will eat what they like and leave the rest.*

Children who *eat* fruit and vegetables *like* fruit and vegetables! This is a hugely crucial factor that will help a child to develop good eating habits – the focus should be on teaching children to like healthy foods, rather than worrying about banning unhealthy things or labelling items as 'bad'.

Children do not miss things if they have not been expected

Ideally, children should grow up being able to eat anything they fancy without having to worry about weight. Indeed there are many people who do just that, tucking into platefuls of food whilst shuddering at the thought of exercise. The simple reason they do not become overweight is that they naturally enjoy a lower-calorie diet without any sense of being deprived. For everyone else, however – those who live for chocolate, would die for a doughnut and pine for pizzas – they either apply restraint against overeating or else suffer the penalty of becoming overweight.

Could a child deprived of cheesecake or chocolate fudge brownies really be happy and fulfilled? Yes! It all depends on expectations. If a person is expecting frequent rich treats then there will be disappointment when they are missing, but if they are not expected then they will not be missed. In the same way most people are not devastated each week when they fail to get the winning numbers in the lottery – they do not really expect to win.

Parents have a big influence on the type, quantity and frequency of family foods, and can improve a child's acceptance of a healthy diet by working on expectations. A child who is used to a healthy diet with only occasional treat items will think that diet is normal – not great, not bad, just normal. But the bonus is that treats will seem far more special than they will to a child who has treats at every meal and in between.

Food does not need to be the centre of life. Despite the attractions of exotic designer menus and the constant supply of tempting new foods, there are plenty of inedible amusements that can fill the 'entertainment gap'. Of course rich foods are there to be enjoyed from time to time, but it is important to get the balance right. In the same way that varying the diet will ensure it is well balanced, varying the way people entertain themselves will help to keep minds and bodies well balanced, by enjoying a mixture of friends, sports, music, films and hobbies, all in addition to good food.

On the other hand, if children are taught the 'entertainment diet' – where food is used for comfort, reward and relief of boredom – then they will be at risk of obesity and all the problems that it brings. The principles in this book can help parents to nurture healthy children who enjoy a wide range of foods (both rich and plain), will tolerate feeling hungry now and again, and who thoroughly enjoy treats and special occasion foods when they are appropriate. Hopefully this will reawaken the novelty and excitement of 'a rare treat'.

Introducing *The Balance of Good Health*: the perfect diet for children

The Balance of Good Health is a simple system that guides the proportions of the five different food groups within a healthy diet. This guide is suitable for children over the age of five, whereas the under-fives may need to eat more fatty or energy-dense foods because of smaller appetites. This is discussed further in Section 2 'Pre-school children'.

Obviously there is no single meal plan that would suit every child, but certain principles apply:

- the diet should be well balanced, and that means varied
- a child's individual needs should be taken into account, as explained in the section below on functional meals
- the diet should be practical, bearing in mind the rest of the family.

What is meant by a 'well-balanced' diet? Too much of some things is just as bad as not enough of others. Without having to read labels or calculate recommended daily allowances (RDAs), it is possible to give a child a well-balanced diet by encouraging as wide a variety of foods as possible. This way the child will get a hotchpotch of all the necessary ingredients whilst avoiding dietary deficiencies that a fussy eater may be susceptible to.

How to use the guide

Figure 1.1 shows what proportions of the five different food groups should appear in the diet over an average day. Roughly a third of mouthfuls (not calories) should come from fruit and vegetables; another third should come from bread, potatoes and cereals, especially wholegrain. The remaining third of the diet should be made up of protein-containing foods, such as meat and fish; dairy products and milk plus a small amount of fatty and sugary foods.

- This balance does not need to be achieved at each meal, but should guide eating throughout the day. So, for example, breakfast consisting of cereals and milk is fine if fruit and vegetables feature in meals and snacks later in the day.
- The guide does not require any calorie counting, but guides what sort of portions should appear on the plate.
- Portion sizes for a particular person tend to be fairly constant – a person who usually has two potatoes is unlikely to suddenly choose five, and so it doesn't matter that the guide does not specify exactly what a portion size is. Details of suitable fruit and vegetable portion sizes for children are described in Chapter 12.
- By getting these proportions roughly right throughout each day, there is no need to worry about individual foods because the overall balance will be good. Eating fatty and sugary foods too frequently will upset the balance, and may mean that healthier parts of the diet are 'pushed off the plate'.
- For foods made up of several ingredients, such as pies, looking at the main listed ingredient will indicate which group it fits best. This will be the first item listed in the ingredients on the packaging. Some foods will fit into two food groups, such as cheesy potato bake. Chapter 13 'The Food Frequency Framework' looks into this in more depth.
- No foods are banned in the guide; if the existing diet contains too much fatty or sugary food, then it can be improved by making those portion sizes smaller or less frequent whilst increasing the number of portions of healthier items.
- The diet will be healthier if there is variety within each food group. For example, eating five portions of carrots each day might provide plenty of vitamin A, but will not supply the full variety of vitamins that a mixture of fruit and vegetables will.
- Although cooking methods are not specified in the guide, it is recommended to use low-fat methods such as grilling rather than frying and to choose lower-fat meat and dairy products on the whole.
- Fruit and vegetables can be fresh, frozen, chilled, canned, dried or served as juice – all will provide an array of vitamins, minerals and fibre.
- Where possible, choosing wholegrain cereals and breads will maximise the amount of micronutrients and fibre in the diet.
- For celebrations, put *The Balance of Good Health* to one side and enjoy whatever is on offer!

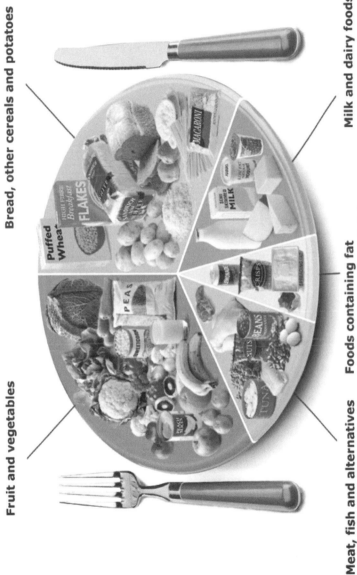

Figure 1.1 *UK National Food Guide: the balance of good health.* Reproduced by kind permission of the Foods Standards Agency.

Putting The Balance of Good Health *into operation*

Simple dietary advice is all very well, but how do parents persuade reluctant children to make changes? And what about parents who feel they eat pretty healthily already and can't understand why their child (or even themselves) may be overweight or have other eating problems? There are many complex factors that govern how and why families eat the way they do and improvements are best if they involve small, gradual changes. Start by making a healthy diet seem relevant and practical, as well as enjoyable.

Children do not need 'special diets', but they will benefit from understanding what makes a normal diet healthy, as well as having confidence in the choices they make. The rest of this chapter looks at how a child builds up a view of a normal diet and how the family affects this. Chapter 2 looks at how flavours and fullness also mould that view.

Functional meals: making food relevant and practical for all the family

Remembering what food does will help in planning well-balanced meals. In addition to the simple joy of eating, food gives energy; the fat layer provides warmth and padding to sit on; vitamins and minerals are needed for growth and to keep brains healthy. But the diet helps many other things too. Fibre is essential for keeping bowels moving; vitamins not only aid seeing in the dark but also are needed for healthy blood and bones; and proteins enable growth and allow the body to repair itself after injury. In essence, the diet allows complex body machinery to work.

Children in particular need plenty of the 'building blocks' part of the diet because they are growing, which means they need plenty of protein, vitamins and minerals to ensure adequate growth. Further details on how diet can boost health and making a good diet seem relevant to junior-aged children are given in Chapter 8 'The healthy body jigsaw'.

Children differ in build, in activity and in preferences and so a perfect diet will need to take all this into account. A very active child will need more calories per day than a less active one, and a higher-protein diet will be indicated if doing rigorous exercise on a regular basis. A skinny child will need fewer calories to tick over than a taller, heavy-boned child. If a child strains uncomfortably on the toilet, a higher-fibre diet will help. A child who is already overweight will be better off eating more fruit and vegetables and fewer high-fat foods, and a child recovering from weight loss will obviously benefit from a high-calorie diet. Illnesses and conditions that require special diets are discussed further in Chapter 15.

The cook in the household will have less work if the same diet suits everyone in the family, rather than have everyone demanding special items. Faddy children can create difficulties purely because they run circles around their parents, even though what they actually eat may still be relatively well balanced. For example, insisting on all ingredients being red or served on separate plates simply isn't practical for most households, so faddy eating tendencies are best nipped in the bud. Behaviour problems that affect eating are covered in

Chapter 6, which looks at how faddy eating can arise and gives ideas on how to deal with fussy eaters.

With the huge pressures on children to eat high-fat, sugary and salty foods, obesity is a risk for more children than ever before, even if they started life as scrawny waifs that had to be coaxed over every mouthful. A well-balanced diet is just as important for slim children as it is for those carrying too much fat. A poor diet that contains too much sugar can lead to tooth decay, abdominal pains and constipation, lethargy and shortage of energy, sugar cravings and mood swings. Children who learn poor eating habits are more likely to develop weight problems in adulthood, even if they were active enough to stay slim in childhood.

A 'perfect' diet is easier to achieve than many parents think because it doesn't need to be perfect at every meal or even every day. The aim is to get the balance of ordinary meals on ordinary days just about right, and to encourage children to eat healthy snacks in addition to the less healthy treats that they love.

Children like to feel they have some control over choice

It is entirely reasonable for parents to feel that they know best for their child. After all, adults are more knowledgeable in general terms, have had more of an education, and have experienced life to a much greater extent than children. In addition, the vast majority of parents want the very best for their children and are prepared to go to great lengths to get things right.

However, children, and especially adolescents, like to annoy, do dangerous or silly things, ignore good advice, take risks, choose dodgy role models to copy and generally do things their own way. Even though adults may know the answer already, children like to find things out for themselves even if that means getting it wrong. It's the process of finding out that makes childhood exciting.

Parents can guide their children successfully but need to understand a few common pitfalls in order to avoid familiar family food fights:

- Studies have shown that the more a parent insists, the more likely a child will resist. When pushing green vegetables it is the parents who cajole the most that end up with the most reluctant children, whereas laid-back parents are more successful.
- Another parent survey showed that 40% of parents actually believe that forbidding their child to eat a certain food will mean the child will stop wanting it. But the opposite is true and banning something makes it more popular – in part by making it appear more intriguing – even if there is a good logical reason for the ban. This same principle has worked well for pop record sales; for example in the 1980s the group Frankie Goes to Hollywood achieved instant success when their record *Relax, Don't Do It* was banned on radio stations due to its dubious messages in the lyrics. If a low-key approach had been taken, the majority of listeners would have remained entirely ignorant of the lyrics, but the ban pushed its profile to such a high level that even uninterested people heard about it.

Does this mean parents can't win? How do parents marry up the opposing factors of knowing what is best but still letting a child make the ultimate choice?

Parents can give children choices whilst still remaining in control

The ultimate way for parents to stay in control is to be certain that children will make the same choices that they would. This requires that the child likes and values the same things as the parent, but children like to do their own experimenting and come to their own decisions. In real life there is no need for children to copy parents exactly as there is usually more than one healthy option. Parents can encourage children to learn healthy principles, so that they are likely to copy general trends and ideas, but at the same time have some flexibility to explore and be different within a safe framework.

The following sections explore how children develop a liking for things, so that parents can influence and guide this process.

Children like things that are familiar

Babies have a natural liking for sweet and salty tastes but dislike sour and bitter flavours. A diet without any sour or bitter elements would be restrictive and bland, so young children learn to like them.

Despite a baby's tendency to spit out new foods, if the food keeps reappearing it becomes familiar so that eventually a baby will accept it. This works more easily if it is cooked or served in a variety of ways, or in combination with other more familiar ingredients. It usually takes anything from five to ten exposures for a new food to become familiar and this principle continues to apply as children grow older. If a carer was unaware of this then a child's reaction to new foods may have been taken at face value and seen as genuine dislike, when it was just an understandable response to something unfamiliar. Even adults can teach themselves to develop a liking for a new food that initially seemed unpleasant by repeatedly trying it, particularly if they see other people enjoying it or appreciate that the food may be healthier. Thus many adults have happily swapped from butter to low-fat spreads and semi-skimmed milk.

Children do as parents do, not as they say (but only up to a point)

Children learn about food in many ways, but sometimes they pick up different messages to the ones intended. Parents are very strong role models, particularly for young children, and if a child is pushed to do something that a parent wouldn't dream of doing then success is unlikely. Telling a child to eat spinach will fall on deaf ears unless other members of the family tuck heartily into it too.

Just as toddlers begin to object to using baby cups and wearing a bib (because no one else around the table is doing so), so they copy everything else that they see, whether it be dipping bread in their soup or demanding pepper on their potatoes. But children's choices are not as simple as copying their parents. Trying to force a child to eat a parental favourite food may encourage deep dislike. This is more of a behavioural matter than anything to do with the food in question; forcing a child to do anything can backfire and produce reluctance rather than enthusiasm. Taking away a child's sense of choice and backing them into a corner is a recipe for war – who will give in first? How angry can the parent become due to a child's refusal to comply? Will the same scene happen next time that food appears? There are many children who learn very early on that they can drive their parents mad over food!

In the same way, forbidding foods makes them more desirable. Unless there is an understandable reason for banning something, such as it being poisonous, then bans merely induce curiosity and make it more intriguing. Children have an innate knack of wanting things that they've been told they shouldn't have. There is no need to forbid foods, but some foods are better reserved for the right time and place.

Once a child has developed a strong liking for, or dislike of, a food then this can be tricky to overrule. The more fuss and attention this preference generates, the more likely it will become entrenched, and so paying little attention is probably a good thing. Exploring ways to broaden the food that a child finds acceptable will increase the overall chance of choosing healthier food because it is liked, not because a parent is pushing it. These methods depend on a child's age and so are dealt with in later age-specific chapters.

Children learn to eat what the family eats

This sounds very obvious, but it is important to get the basics right because patterns learned in childhood will often stay for life. If rich fatty foods are served on a daily basis then this will be normal, familiar and hence liked by the children in the household. If parents puts vegetables onto everyone's plate apart from their own, it won't be long before children begin to question this and then to copy not eating vegetables too.

Government advice clearly recommends five portions of fruit and vegetables every day for everyone, as a minimum. But if no one in the family eats more than two portions on average, then children in that household will do the same. Just telling them to eat more won't help unless the family go for the same trend.

Sharon was fed up with throwing away good food. After her seven-year-old daughter, Holly, had had trouble with tummy ache and time off school, the school nurse suggested some dietary changes that included more fruit and vegetables. Sharon found grapes were expensive, but this was the only fruit Holly would eat. She had cooked endless platefuls of carrots and broccoli only to throw most of it away. When she saw the nurse again she complained about how difficult it was to get Holly to eat fresh produce at all.

'Well I've seen her tucking into apples at school, and pears,' replied the nurse, 'because I sometimes supervise break time and they all get a portion of fruit then. Which is your favourite fruit or veg?'

Sharon looked surprised and then a little embarrassed. 'Well I don't eat them myself, except for peas and bananas. But I've told Holly she's got to eat them.'

The nurse suggested that Holly might be copying those around her, so she would do as friends did at school, but at home she copied her mum by refusing to eat them. Sharon could see that perhaps her own diet could be improved and this might encourage Holly too.

These common patterns of how the family eats teach children to put food in some sort of order or 'food hierarchy'. They work out which are common daily filling foods, which are reserved for occasional treats and which foods their parents dislike. This effect is very important for communities that eat hot or spicy foods. Asian children are not born liking spicy curries, but watching the rest of the household enjoy hot foods encourages them to accept these foods themselves.

If parents enjoy fresh produce and serve it regularly then children will grow up assuming it forms part of the common daily filling foods (also known as the staple diet), even if the type of produce varies from day to day. If parents won't touch a courgette with a curtain pole then it is no wonder that their children wrinkle their noses at greens.

For sugary or fatty foods the same applies. If they are served up at every meal then children assume they are the mainstay of a normal diet. Some parents may comment at how wonderful the pudding is in an attempt to make the food seem special, but if it still turns up regularly then children will see it as a daily food.

Children also learn from eating away from home

Children have a keen eye for what goes on around them, particularly if they are watching other children enjoy themselves. Meals at friends' houses, nursery, school or other relatives' houses are learning experiences and a time to weigh up how other people eat.

In a group of pre-school children who didn't like vegetables, researchers were able to show that these children began to choose vegetables after they had watched other children at the nursery do so. Their desire to copy what the other children did was stronger than their uncertainty about vegetables. In this situation it would be a shame if a parent unknowingly reminded such a child that he 'didn't like' a food that he was actually starting to tolerate or even enjoy. Better to assume that all foods can be eaten by anyone, and, if in doubt, keep portions very small.

Some parents can list half a dozen foods that their child 'hates', but a true dislike of a food is fairly uncommon and children are really stating that the food is strange, rather than offensive. 'Hated' foods may be eaten without any fuss if there is suitable distraction by, for example, a special occasion.

Jacob went to tea at his friend Kyle's house. After a riotous game trashing Kyle's bedroom, the two nine-year-olds and Kyle's older sister all tucked heartily into a plate of lasagne and had a competition to see how many slices of cucumber they could push onto their little fingers. Jacob ate well over half of what was on his plate before saying he had had enough.

Later, when his mum came to collect him, she apologised for Jacob's poor appetite. 'He eats like a sparrow at home; I hope he didn't waste too much.'

Kyle's mum shook her head. 'He ate just as much as the others; they love lasagne.'

'Lasagne?' said Jacob's mum in disbelief. 'I can only get him to eat plain pasta at home without any sauce at all.'

'Well, they were so busy destroying the cucumber I don't think they gave it much thought.'

Alternatively, simple perseverance can work if the food keeps reappearing in different forms without discussion, so that eventually it appears familiar. Sometimes, however, it will be evident that children know their own minds and have a genuine dislike. Remind them that tastes may change as they get older and leave it at that.

Children will learn from dieting behaviours in adults

When adults 'go on a diet' they tend to eat differently from the rest of the household and make numerous remarks such as 'I'm not allowed that' or 'I shouldn't'. This dietary restraint is actually associated with greater feelings of hunger and a strong sense of denial. It is also often associated with feeling moody and is definitely linked to guilt when forbidden foods are eaten. Girls in particular are sensitive to copying dieting behaviour that they see around them, and even if they do not apply much restraint they may still develop a sense of guilt about eating enjoyable food.

If a parent is trying to diet then children will benefit from hearing positive comments about the healthy things that the diet recommends, rather than sensing how much the parent misses what seem to be the good things in life. If fruit and vegetables form a significant part of the diet, make sure they are served to the whole household. Healthy eating is not only for people who want to lose weight.

Why do families eat what they eat?

So far, we have seen that children tend to eat what they like, and they tend to like what is familiar, but they will object to things that are forced on them. In order to get children to choose healthy eating patterns throughout their lives, it will help to see their family set an example. This is more straightforward after understanding where family eating tendencies come from. Some factors will influence the choice of particular foods, whilst other factors will influence eating behaviour.

How does eating food differ from eating a meal?

Mealtimes are social occasions and children will take in far more than just the calories on their plate. Family meals are a time for catching up on gossip, checking general behaviour and teaching manners, sharing worries and keeping the whole family working as a team.

Eating food alone, or in a distracted setting such as in front of the television, will create different influences. These settings are commonly times when people eat out of boredom or for entertainment, rather than in response to hunger. Hence, fullness cues may be overridden because eating is such a reliable way to create that feel-good factor and can temporarily blot out a sense of loneliness or boredom. Eating small mouthfuls over a prolonged period (such as snacking in front of a film) means that insufficient food will be in the stomach at any one time to create a feeling of fullness. Both may result in overeating. These factors are discussed more in Chapter 2.

If children like to snack in front of the television, remember the laziness factor. They are more likely to snack on something that is easily to hand than to get up and find a choice snack, so put fruit or a dish of raisins by the sofa. (And don't forget to grumble when they've eaten it all, because kids get a kick out of doing things they're not supposed to do!)

How do household traditions take shape?

Most families will have a selection of traditions that they follow, for example eating fish on Fridays, having Yorkshire pudding with roast beef, combining beef burgers with chips or sausages with mash, and eating roast dinner on Sundays and leftovers on Mondays. Many of these traditions reflect society and happen in most households, but some will be very specific to each family, having been handed down through generations, such as what favourite pudding will accompany a special occasion or what cold remedy is first choice for winter sniffles. These traditions travel from grandparents down to parents and will continue into the next generation's home, with small modifications along the way. They will be shaped by personal choice, advertising, genes, the pressures on lifestyle and pester power from kids.

Traditions that go unquestioned can be very useful, for example that two pieces of toast make an adequate lunch. This takes away the 'how much do I eat' question, replacing it with a simple habit. Some traditions, however, can do the opposite if they lead to unhealthy eating patterns going unquestioned. For example, if it is a family habit to go out for fish and chips on a Friday evening, this may become an issue if oven chips and other fried bits for kids appear most other evenings of the week, so that fried foods are being served most days.

Consider ways to modify any traditions that are creating problems. Question why the same foods are purchased every week. Is it time to forget fixed ideas about what foods should go with what? Is there any reason why a burger must be accompanied by chips? Why not a jacket potato or new potatoes with a knob of butter and some tomato salsa? What about sausages and rice? Or fish fingers and pasta? By questioning the way that ingredients are put together on a plate, a child can be introduced to variety more easily. This is a safer start than introducing new foods and flavours together.

Convenience foods have limitations

Lifestyle pressures are becoming greater for many parents, with time at an absolute premium. Cooking the traditional 'meat and two veg' requires preparation time as well as eating time and that is often simply not practical. For working parents and for families where the kids have school clubs and sports fixtures most days of the week, time just to sit down as a family can be rare. The food industry has recognised this and provides ready-meals of every size and variety, which has led to a new food category – 'convenience foods'.

Whilst these convenience foods help in one way, they take away a parent's ability to decide on the specific ingredients of a meal or the portion sizes, and they take away the need to sit down as a family. It is easier to serve ready-meals one by one as they come out of the microwave, leading to the phrase 'TV dinners' as members of the family can be distracted whilst each portion arrives. Distraction by the television also stops a child focusing on when they feel full, leaving the temptation to eat until all the food has disappeared.

Convenience foods are popular, particularly with children, because they are designed to be tasty. This usually means they have a high salt and saturated fat content and are low in vitamins and fibre. Of course it is possible to bolster the packaged food with some fresh produce, but this reduces the convenience factor. Serving these meals on a regular basis will teach children that they are common basic foods, and so they will choose them themselves as they grow up. Families wishing to find convenient alternatives to 'convenience foods' could try cooking double quantities when there *is* time to cook and then freezing half. This allows them to stay in control of both the nutritional content of the food and portion size.

Some ideas for convenience foods are given in the Food Frequency Framework in Chapter 13, but there are also many cookbooks available that give suggestions for quick healthy meals that require little more than throwing ingredients onto a plate and pressing the 'on' button of the microwave (*see* Appendix 2).

Should children eat 'children's food'?

Another threat to healthy household traditions over the last few decades has been the emergence of another new food category – 'children's food' – and this has been a major factor in the increasing levels of obesity in our children today.

Years ago, children would eat the same things that their parents ate. As people began to eat out more often, pubs and restaurants recognised that they would do better trade if they catered for children as well as adults, particularly if the children's menu was cheaper. The 'children's menu' is now found in most eating places, offering simple fail-safe foods that most children will eat. However, this means almost exclusively fried salty foods, with a virtual absence of fruit and vegetables altogether. Most items are batter coated, containing processed meat or fish with a high fat content.

Whilst this is fine for an occasional meal, the concept of 'children's food' has crept into the general approach to feeding children so that now the average child eats chips or fried food several times a week and is unlikely to eat more than two portions of fruit and vegetables per day, compared to the recommended five. One in five children in a recent survey ate no fruit at all and less than half of them ate leafy green vegetables.

Once again, 'children's food' tends to be convenient, with fried bits from the freezer easily heated up, so it is now commonplace in the home as well as in restaurants. School dinners followed suit after minimum nutritional guidelines were removed in the late 1970s, but happily nutritional standards have been reinstated in the last few years, which, along with the current high media interest in school meals, has led to healthy school meal initiatives being put into place. Serving 'children's food' to children on a regular basis is a problem because:

- children will develop a taste for fried and salty foods
- fresh produce may seem bland and boring in comparison
- the convenience factor may make the effort of preparing traditional food seem more trouble than it is worth, particularly if children are reluctant to eat it
- children will be less tolerant of eating a wide variety of foods, which is necessary for a well-balanced diet.

It is best if they can be reserved for occasional meals when the convenience factor is really useful. Instead, explore easy-to-prepare convenience foods that have a better nutritional balance.

Parents can make their wishes known

Food manufacturers will continue to produce and market convenience products because there will always be some people who will continue to buy them, but restaurants and pubs are more sensitive to customer demand. If more and more parents ask for healthier options on children's menus (such as fresh vegetables or salad with burger and chips, or plates of pasta, or simply half-portions of adult foods) then these food outlets may once again lead the way. At the time of writing burger chains are currently getting this message.

Celebratory foods are special

With heavy marketing of endless varieties of new foods, it is now common for families to eat rich and interesting foods on a regular basis. In bygone days, a party was a time for going to extra lengths to prepare special foods. Nowadays, these can be purchased fairly cheaply and ready prepared, so that cost and trouble are no longer an issue. So what now distinguishes a normal food from a celebratory food? For children's parties there is little difference. Take-out cartons from a burger chain or pizza parlour are popular, but these feature as part of many children's regular meals too.

One odd factor that frequently distinguishes celebratory food is guilt! Nowadays, although people are encouraged to buy rich, high-fat and high-sugar foods on a regular basis by the marketing of these products, they sense that they are not healthy. Because there is no obvious mechanism to limit how often these foods are eaten (because they are no longer particularly expensive and someone else has gone to the trouble of preparing them), it means that many people eat them too frequently. And when people try to apply restraint this results in the food appearing even more attractive. The more people agonise over 'should I/ shouldn't I', the more guilty they feel if they then give in.

One solution to reduce this problem is to put in place clear family guidelines as to when rich foods are appropriate. This forms the basis of the Food Frequency Framework (*see* Chapter 13), which offers guidance on which foods are suitable for daily, weekly or rare occasion consumption. By teaching these rules to children they will feel happier about eating ordinary foods on ordinary days, without any sense of missing out as rich foods were not expected. It will boost confidence about declining delicious foods in the wrong situation, but will also enhance a thorough enjoyment of eating treats when the situation is right without a trace of guilt.

Accessible food gets eaten

Food accessibility and availability is a reason for many food choices and is a current hot topic in the media. Everyone knows that burger and chips won't feature on a Weight Watcher's diet sheet, yet burger bars are on every street corner. If they're so bad then why doesn't the Government ban them?

It all comes down to personal choice. The food industry will say that they are providing what people want – and they're busy enough to prove it! But on street corners there are no real alternatives to burgers – apart from pizzas, fish and chips, or deep-fried chicken. Is this array of fried and processed foods giving real choice? What about healthy fast food choices?

It is a vicious circle. People buy burgers because they are easily accessible, so the food industry provides more of them, saying that that is what the public wants. The food industry is making a killing (quite literally) from putting convenience foods in every nook and cranny, in the name of consumer choice. ('No one is forcing people to buy my chocolate bars' responds the marketing executive, smugly.) But there is only a choice of unhealthy options. There is no basket of fruit at the till in the garden centre, but there are at least 30 types of confectionery on sale, when all that was needed was a bag of soil and a garden gnome. And has anyone ever seen boiled potatoes in a chip shop?

There are changes afoot with more sandwich and salad bar outlets and the occasional 'healthy' item on sale in burger bars, yet there is a very long way to go: convenience foods need further improvements to their high fat, salt and sugar content as well as more choice of wholegrain and fresh produce in order to fit into a well-balanced diet.

If children are to eat fruit and vegetables then they need to be put in reach: stick them in coat pockets, leave a bag of apples in the car, put them into lunch boxes, pop sliced carrots into hungry mouths whilst preparing tea, hand them out at the drop of a hat. Banish that old image of the untouched fruit bowl with its few shrivelled apples!

Summary points

- Childhood lasts a long time. There is time to get it wrong then try again another day.
- Teach children to enjoy healthy foods rather than worry about banning less healthy things.
- Question which household traditions are worth hanging on to and prioritise family meals.
- Avoid too many 'convenience' or 'children's' foods and make sure celebratory foods are appropriate to avoid feelings of guilt.
- Make good choice seem relevant, but be clear that there is a choice or behaviour battles will result.
- Ensure a parent's example doesn't encourage poor choices: parents should do what they say themselves and be aware that their dieting behaviour will influence children.
- Keep the decision-making process low-key because too much agonising over one issue will create ideas for winding up a parent.
- Have faith both in the child and the normal mechanisms by which children learn. Even rebellious kids bent on a course of self-destruction come through difficult phases if given a bit of time and space to experiment.

Chapter 2

Flavours and fullness

Flavours: there's no accounting for taste – or is there?

Flavour is an important aspect of food. For a start, if food didn't appeal then eating would be a chore. In addition to flavour, the texture, moisture content, temperature and freshness of foods all play a part in how appealing a food is.

Flavours colour eating habits in two distinct ways: firstly via hunger factors, such as the filling power and satisfaction produced by a food, and secondly via emotional factors, which means the associations that food has with other aspects of life.

Early experience of flavours is important

As a general rule, it is easier to provide a well-balanced diet if a child likes a wide variety of foods.

Whether a baby was breast- or bottle-fed is the first thing that affects a child's tolerance of new foods. Bottle or formula milk always tastes the same, but breast milk varies in flavour according to what the mother herself has been eating (*see* Box 2.1). Research suggests that breast-fed babies find it easier than bottle-fed babies to accept new flavours when solids are introduced.

Box 2.1 Why should breast milk vary in flavour?

The taste of breast milk varies according to what the mother has been eating. If she eats a diet full of garlic or vanilla, for example, she will produce more strongly flavoured milk than if she ate a bland diet. Studies have shown that the length of time that a baby suckles at the breast increases when the mother eats strong flavours, but decreases when she sticks to a bland diet, suggesting that babies like variations in flavour. This is helpful to babies because if the mother lives in a community where spicy food is eaten frequently, then her flavoured milk will mean her baby will be better prepared to accept spicy foods during the weaning process.

From eight to 12 months of age, babies are open to all things new. This 'food window' provides the opportunity to try as many new flavours and textures as possible, and the more a baby experiences at this stage the less likely fussy eating will develop. By getting used to different flavours children also get used to the idea of variety itself and so learn to tolerate not knowing what is coming next. Hence pureeing all the things that the rest of the household eats is preferable to jars of bland baby foods.

Chapter 4 takes a more detailed look at weaning and feeding pre-school children.

Why do children like chocolate?

The majority of children love chocolate and this fondness usually starts very early on. Children will develop a taste for any food that stops them feeling bored and hungry, which explains why crisps and chocolate, which are handed out frequently in between meals, are popular. If chocolate were only served at the end of meals, when a child was less hungry, it would be far less appealing, but it doesn't usually feature as part of a normal meal. The more often children eat tasty, high-calorie foods when really hungry or thoroughly bored, the more satisfying the food will appear.

If the chocolate is also nicely packaged in interesting child-sized shapes, perhaps with an accompanying toy or familiar cartoon picture, the more its flavour will be linked with feeling happy, contented and having fun. Its effect on taking away hunger is now intermingled with its ability to entertain.

However, any food can achieve the same popularity – it requires planning snacks with a little care, so that healthy foods are to hand when out and about with a fractious child in a pushchair. Parents can grab the opportunity of a bored and hungry child to offer foods they want their child to eat, such as fresh or dried fruit, bread sticks, lumps of cheese or sliced raw vegetables. As long as the child was not expecting something specific, such as chocolate, then any of these foods can relieve both boredom and hunger.

Charlie, a busy three-year old, didn't usually eat much at mealtimes and tended to get hungry in between meals. His mum would often give him a chocolate snack at this point, partly because he saw his older sisters snacking on chocolate and wanted what they had, but also because she knew it would taste delicious, stop him feeling hungry and was a convenient snack to carry around. Charlie soon learned to link the flavour of chocolate with tasting good and feeling better, plus it was interesting to play with. He didn't mind what form the chocolate was in, whether biscuits, ice cream or milk shakes, it was the flavour that he liked.

If Charlie was given chocolate at the end of a meal, even if he was already full, his liking for it was stronger than the discomfort of eating too much, and so chocolate would always be eaten whenever it was on offer.

Another three-year old, Freddie, was only offered chocolate at the end of meals, when he was already feeling full. In between meals, his mum gave him pieces of fruit in a little tub or packets of raisins or sometimes a sandwich or breadsticks. He wasn't usually interested in chocolate at the end of his meals and he didn't like chocolate milk shake, although he quite liked licking the chocolate off biscuits before he ate them. He had made no strong links with the flavour of chocolate, other than possibly associating it with being bloated and perhaps feeling a bit sick.

However, once Freddie started nursery, he was given chocolate snacks in between meals when he was hungry and it wasn't long before he began to like it. But, when he is hungry at home, he is just as happy being given fruit or a sandwich or chocolate or a packet of crisps, because all these flavours have given him a feel-good factor in the past.

For some children (and some adults) the feel-good factor from chocolate may become strong enough to make any meal feel incomplete without a bit of chocolate at the end, regardless of the size of the meal. This is the start of a food craving. Eating to satisfy a food craving will easily outweigh a sense of fullness, because food cravings are driven by the intense pleasure associated with a flavour, rather than eating in response to feeling hungry.

What does a flavour say about a food?

People have a good memory for flavours. This is a protective mechanism so that if a poisonous food was eaten or if bad food caused illness, then it will be recognised quickly if that food is encountered again. This mechanism is sometimes the reason for a strong childhood dislike of a food if an illness coincided with eating a particular flavour, which then became imprinted in the memory as one to avoid. The specific food may not have caused the illness itself, but because the illness came on soon after it was eaten, the association was made.

Flavours and the smell of a food are good at indicating food quality – whether it is rich and sickly, so not to be overeaten, or bland and mild, or sometimes whether food is going off. It is not simply flavour that shows this, the fat and sugar or salt content is important in working this out, but flavour counts for some of it.

Flavour can be overridden by advertising and packaging

Whether a food is popular depends on all sorts of things alongside its taste. Having tried some of the children's foods currently available in shops and restaurants, it is obvious that some manufacturers are not relying solely on flavour for people to come back for more.

Food packaging makes a huge difference to the impression a food creates. Food is fashionable and many people like to try new food crazes, cooking techniques or a new restaurant, all of which may change acceptance of flavours. Heavy food advertising and marketing create a confusing picture of what is healthy when walking around a supermarket and health messages sometimes add to a food's appeal. Television advertising has an especially powerful effect to make children want certain foods, with research clearly showing that the frequency of children demanding unhealthy snacks is directly related to how often they appear on television.

However, families can help children to learn to question advertising tactics by discussing whether they think a particular product matched its advertising claims. It is healthy for children to learn a bit of cynicism early on, rather than be taken for a ride too often. Ways to make children more aware of gimmicks and marketing tricks are covered in later age-related chapters.

People can be surprisingly emotional about food

That is not to say that candyfloss might make someone burst into tears, but people are sensitive to the way emotions are linked to certain foods. The commonest example is using food as a reward, but it is also used for bribery, for comfort and for punishment. All of these issues have an effect on whether certain foods are loved or hated, high profile or just off the menu.

> Oliver, at six years of age, struggled with his handwriting, but since starting in his new class he worked extremely hard and at the end of term was given a certificate for effort. With the certificate came a packet of sherbet fizz sweets.
>
> 'Well done, Oliver,' said his mum, as he presented the certificate to her at home time. 'Shall we swap the sherbet sweets for something else when we get home, because you don't like them, do you?'
>
> Oliver gave her a startled look and charged off to play with his friends, taking the sweets with him. These were highly coveted rewards in that playground, and he was going to be seen eating them regardless of how they tasted!

Children learn to like things that are generally highly valued, and soon realise that possession is the important factor, not necessarily the eating of the prize. Prizes are all the more desirable if they are in very short supply, whereas if every child were regularly guaranteed the same prize then it would no longer be special or worth coveting. This aspect of 'treats' for children is sometimes forgotten. If chocolate orange segments are given out every day then they are not a treat, but a basic foodstuff. A treat is something out of the ordinary.

Using food for punishment can create problems. Parents may be tempted to ban a popular item because of poor behaviour, but this will make that food more in demand and may encourage a child to overeat it when it is available. On the other hand, banning an unpopular food wouldn't be much of a penalty. Where possible it is better to see food as nutrition rather than as a means of controlling a child's behaviour, or the child's view of food will become muddled.

Fullness – the hidden switch within

Recognising the sensation of fullness is one of the most valuable areas to explore if children are to avoid obesity in the future. Studies suggest that overweight people have poorer 'fullness' cues than people of normal weight, which may partly explain why they eat more than they need. There are many reasons for this tendency, a particular one being the amount of mealtime coaxing by a parent. Rather than helping, parents who try to control what and how much their children eat end up with children who show the least ability to regulate their eating when not with their parents.

It is important to allow children to tune in to their own signals that say when to stop eating, rather than a parent taking over control of what is eaten. Parents may not always be present, in which case how will the child know when to stop eating? And how aware are parents of how hungry the child is or what his energy requirements are that day? Energy requirements vary according to how quickly a child is growing, what food was eaten earlier, whether the child has been charging around or taking things easy, and whether extra calories have been consumed that day in the form of drinks or snacks. A child is in the best position to know all this and has an inbuilt mechanism to recognise it – hunger – if allowed to use it.

Babies have an inbuilt mechanism to know when they are full

Tiny babies have a primitive cycle of hunger stimulating crying, which then promotes being fed by the mother, which produces the reassuring sensation of feeling full, so that the baby begins to settle (*see* Figure 2.1). This is the first real lesson learned by a baby; after drinking milk, the sensation of hunger goes away and is replaced by feeling full, which is more pleasurable than hunger. Babies have a natural ability to recognise when they are full and so know when to stop feeding.

A breast-feeding mother will have little idea of the exact quantity her baby has had, and will generally rely on her baby to take enough. She will have an idea of this by how quickly the baby settles after a feed and how soon the next feed is needed. Good growth is another extremely reassuring way of assessing how much milk has been taken, even though this information is not available at the end of each feed. As feeding becomes established, a breast-feeding mother will also recognise how engorged her breasts feel before and after a feed.

For bottle-fed babies the situation is different because there is far more scope for parents to control how much milk is taken. The quantity taken is easily measured and often generates more worry than reassurance, sometimes being noted down and compared with other new babies of the same age, which generates yet more worry. Mothers are designed to worry over their children, and milk intake is one of the commonest things that raise concern.

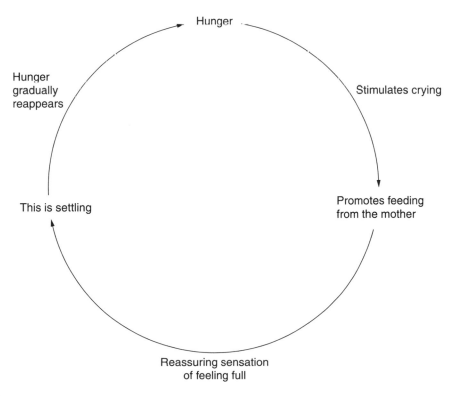

Figure 2.1

A drawback of bottle-feeding is that a parent can override their baby's natural fullness signal by persisting with a feed, waking the baby as he or she nods off half way through the bottle, and generally encouraging all that was prepared to be finished up. Whilst it may reassure an anxious parent to know that a good feed was taken, the baby is already learning to ignore his or her own fullness cues and comply with what the mother wants.

Babies sense how filling their milk is

Studies have shown that a baby can adjust the volume of milk taken according to its energy content. In other words, if a baby is given a watery feed then more will be drunk compared to a more concentrated feed. Babies also take in more milk if thirsty and in need of more fluids, such as in hot weather. Breast milk, miraculously, will alter according to such factors as the weather, and a mother will produce weaker milk in hot dry weather, so her baby is able to take in more liquid for the same amount of energy to avoid dehydration. Formula milk will only vary if it is prepared differently.

The process by which babies self-regulate their milk intake goes on during each feed as well as over a 24-hour period. So, a baby may take a small feed at one time, but make up for it with a larger feed later on. The more babies are encouraged to finish up bottles and to stick rigidly to four-hourly feeds, the harder it will be for their natural feedback mechanism to work, meaning that their inbuilt fullness cues may already be pushed to one side. Demand feeding is a preferable plan, allowing a baby to feed when hungry and to stop when full. Whilst parents may initially worry that demand feeding will create a fusspot whose mother is constantly at baby's beck and call, demand-fed babies are just as likely to settle nicely into a predictable routine as when feeds are carefully timed.

Further hints for confident and successful breast and bottle-feeding are given in Chapter 4.

Older children regulate their intake over the whole day, rather than at each meal, too

Left to their own devices children will eat roughly the amount they want over a 24-hour period, even if they seem to eat next to nothing at mealtimes. It is far easier for a child to plan how much to eat at any time if meals usually follow a set pattern or if that day's menu is clear at the start of the meal. A child will be prone to overeating if a favourite pudding arrives unexpectedly following a large and tasty main course. If there is some warning about what is for afters then a child will be able to save some room.

As children get older, eating patterns can remain a source of constant worry, progressing, for some children, from simple faddy eating to complex behaviour problems, particularly if a child learns how much they can fox and manipulate well-meaning parents at mealtimes.

Behaviour problems and normal growth patterns for younger children are discussed in Chapter 6, but Box 2.2 lists some guiding principles to be aware of.

Box 2.2 A child's growth is more informative than eating tendency

- Smaller children will have smaller appetites.
- Children who grow well may appear to eat like sparrows.
- Children who grow well are allowed to eat like sparrows!
- If concerned, monitor food intake over 24 hours rather than just at mealtimes, as snacks and extras may make up a sizeable portion of a child's daily intake.
- Fusspot phases usually pass if little attention is paid.
- Children will rarely starve themselves out of choice. If a child's growth pattern has changed then look for a reason.
- If a child starts out on the lowest growth line, it is expected that they will follow that same line as time goes by.
- A child's growth pattern will sometimes cross one of the centile lines, but if it crosses two centile lines then this should be looked into. If there are concerns that a child is failing to thrive, this can be discussed with a health visitor or family doctor, in order for the child's growth to be monitored.

Should a child be encouraged to clear the plate?

One longstanding issue at mealtimes is whether children should be encouraged to finish up everything on their plate. This is commonly a learned behaviour: people tend to encourage their children to do so if that is how their own parents wanted things when they were younger. There are many reasons for feeling it is good parenting to encourage children to do this (*see* Box 2.3).

Box 2.3 Reasons why parents justify encouraging a child to eat

- It is wasteful to leave good food.
- How can we leave good food to waste when there are millions starving in Africa?
- Some people feel it is impolite to leave food uneaten.
- If a child fills up at mealtimes, there may be less chance of wanting snacks later on.
- If a child has been told to eat up during a meal, the parent may feel justified in refusing snacks later.
- If the child has to eat up everything on the plate then perhaps healthy items will be consumed in the process, whereas if the child has choice about what is eaten, won't the vegetables be left out altogether?

By looking at these reasons from the child's viewpoint, it is possible to come to very different conclusions. The following section takes each reason in turn.

Is it wasteful for a child to leave good food?

No. The person who prepared and served the meal is responsible for the amount that was cooked and the amount that was served. Unless a child saved up money, worked out the menu ingredients, did the shopping and then prepared the meal, there will be no sense of what wasting food means. As far as the child is concerned hunger meant eating and then fullness meant it was time to stop. The quantity of food purchased, prepared and served was not the child's responsibility, and so neither was the amount left over at the end of the meal.

One solution to the difficulty of portion sizes for children is to allow each child to serve their own portion from the table, or to ask how much of each item is wanted. If a child has chosen a certain amount, then it would be more reasonable to expect it to be eaten. If children appear to have eyes bigger than their stomachs they can be encouraged to take a smaller amount to begin with, and ask for a second helping if still hungry.

Will it help starving nations if we avoid food wastage in this country?

It is sad that food availability is so uneven throughout the world, but encouraging a child in western leafy suburbia to overeat when already full will merely increase the risk of obesity. By encouraging children to override their own 'fullness' cues, the most reliable mechanism that children have for eating sensibly will be destroyed. Factors that encourage obesity in one country will have no benefit on food shortages elsewhere.

The most positive way to reduce food wastage is to review the amount of food prepared and served. If the family are regularly leaving food untouched because they feel full, then too much food is being prepared. Preparing too little will be safer than too much, as the meal can always be padded out with bread or pudding etc. if quantities were significantly underestimated. If excess food is prepared then find out ways to use up leftovers at the next meal.

Leaving food might be seen as impolite

If a person has been brought up to feel that leaving food is impolite, this can be addressed by allowing children to serve themselves, but with the advice that if they have asked for or taken something then it is polite to finish it, as above. In addition, children can be taught to pay attention whilst a meal is being served so they can express their views on how much they want. Parents might allow untouched food to be returned to the serving dish if a child realises he has taken too much.

Make sure children are confident enough to ask for small portions or to say 'no' to new things at mealtimes if they are not sure when visiting friends' houses. Explain that if they feel really full, they can be excused from eating more after asking politely to leave what is left.

Will eating well at mealtimes reduce the chance of snacking later?

If a child eats until they are full, they will be no more likely to snack later than if they had overeaten at the meal. In fact, as discussed above, if children have been taught to ignore their inner messages about being full, they will be more likely to snack following a large meal out of either boredom or habit, because the awareness of when they are full has been lost.

It is questionable whether snacking should be seen as a problem at all. Other omnivores such as monkeys tend to graze on food throughout the day, rather than sticking to set mealtimes. Rigid mealtimes are generated by society and are not a natural tendency, so perhaps it is understandable for children to want to eat when hungry, rather than because the clock is chiming mealtime. In our society it is more convenient for children to fit in with set mealtimes, because schools and workplaces follow the clock. But there are no fixed rights and wrongs about this, and it is up to individual families to decide when snacks are suitable. However, the type of snack is important, and this is discussed in the nutrition section later in the book.

Will insisting on a clean plate mean healthy food gets eaten?

It would be nice to think so, but as discussed at the start of this chapter, children will object to things that are forced on them. Bribing them to clear their plate by offering an unhealthy but desirable pudding will raise the pudding's profile, so increasing the chance of developing a sweet tooth, because children grow to like foods that are used as a reward. It may also encourage them to ignore when they are full. Instead, remember that healthy eating involves children choosing for themselves. If a child is taught to enjoy healthy foods there won't be a problem.

How can a parent balance staying in control with letting a child eat what they want?

This is easier than it sounds. The process of putting a child in charge doesn't mean that parents lose all influence. First, parents have control over what options a child can choose from. A parent might suggest choosing two vegetables from a list, or that the child decides how they are cooked or whether eaten raw, or that there is a choice of whether to eat fruit after lunch or after tea, or perhaps as a mid-afternoon snack. Avoid suggesting options such as 'would you like boiled potatoes or chips?' or progress will be slow. If a family is aiming to reduce how often chips are served, a child can still have some say in this by being involved in such questions as 'shall we have chips on Thursday or at the weekend?' or 'should we have our "chips night" with a burger and salad this week or with broccoli and ham?'

Secondly, a parent and child can discuss the child's choices together in order to find out if they were good or not. Commenting in an explanatory way without being critical will help children consider different choices next time the situation arises. Box 2.4 provides examples of this.

Box 2.4 Examples of commenting in an explanatory way to help children consider different choices

Emily took too much on her plate

- Discuss why this might matter.

- Perhaps someone else at the table had less than their share.
- Rather than having to throw food away at the end of a meal, it is better to ask for a small portion and then ask for more if still hungry; leftover food can be put in the fridge for another day if it has not been touched.
- If she fills up too soon then she won't have room for the rest of the meal.
- Even if a favourite food is on the table, it is not an excuse for overeating. Instead savour each mouthful by eating the favourite food more slowly.

Brandon took too much, but then ate it all

- Discuss some of the problems of overeating.
- It feels great to really tuck in now and then, but it is best not to do so too often or people run the risk of becoming overweight. Being overweight can lead to illnesses and health problems.
- Overeating causes an unpleasant sensation of feeling bloated and uncomfortable.
- Explain how eating food more slowly can be more enjoyable, with less risk of overeating.
- Make sure a child knows that they may leave food on their plate if they have had enough.
- For a child who is prone to eating anything in front of them, ask them during the meal whether they are starting to feel full and to think about when they have had enough, rather than letting them assume that the meal only ends when all the food has vanished.

Alisha chose a disgusting-looking cake in the bakery

- Even though the cake was beautifully decorated it was obviously going to taste sickly and horrid. Discuss how appearances can be misleading and that sometimes the plain-looking things in life are the tastiest.
- Explain that sometimes it is fun to choose something because it looks pretty even if it doesn't taste great, and in that case there is no need to eat it all – the fun was in its appearance, it was not being purchased for the sake of nutrition.
- Avoid giving the child a hard time if she leaves most of it.

George insisted on a huge cream puff covered in chocolate

- Discuss whether a special food such as this is suitable for every day, for occasional meals or for celebrations.
- Even though it looks interesting and may taste delicious, it is the sort of food that tastes best when reserved for special occasions like parties or Christmas. If rich foods are eaten often then there will be nothing exciting to celebrate with – celebratory foods will seem ordinary and boring.
- Eating too much cream and chocolate causes weight problems, so these foods are best reserved for occasional days. Then, when the occasion is right, they can be enjoyed right down to the last crumb.

Summary points

Flavours

- Encouraging children to eat a wide variety of foods will make it easier to provide a well-balanced diet.
- When children are feeling very hungry in between meals, offer varied and unpredictable snacks that include plain foods and fruit and vegetables. This will help children to appreciate healthy foods and prevent them from getting hooked on crisps and chocolate.
- Chocolate and crisps can form part of a balanced diet if they are served during meals, rather than only when a child is very bored and hungry.
- Be wary of making children covet unhealthy treats by using them for bribery and as rewards.

Fullness

- Teach children to recognise and be aware of when they are full.
- Remember that children regulate how much they eat over a 24-hour period, rather than at each meal.
- Review family approaches to whether a child is encouraged to finish food on the plate.
- Explore practical ways for children to eat sensibly, without having to throw food away after each meal.
- Children can be given plenty of freedom to make their own choices whilst parents remain in overall control.

Chapter 3

Measuring a child's size and boosting activity

Any child who eats lots of snacks as well as high-calorie main meals will need to do plenty of exercise to burn off the calories or run the risk of storing these surplus calories as fat. With the huge change in children's diets over the last 50 years, increasing numbers of children are becoming overweight, even though they may be active and busy. Parents are advised to monitor their child's height and weight from time to time to check if growth is healthy.

If there is concern about a child being overweight then a good place to start is by assessing activity levels to get an idea as to whether changing exercise patterns will be enough to improve things, or whether there will need to be changes to the diet too. For most children there may be room to improve both aspects of life, whereas for very busy children, looking at eating patterns may be the most fruitful place to start.

Measuring a child's size

Monitoring growth using growth charts

The best way to monitor a child's growth is by taking occasional height and weight measurements and plotting them on a growth chart. Do not be alarmed by a one-off measurement that seems not to have followed the trend. It may be explained by a different person having taken the measurement or because the child wriggled at a crucial moment, giving an inaccurate reading. Several readings taken over a space of time will give a better idea of the trend, which is more useful.

When looking at a growth chart, whether for weight or for height, there will be a series of centile lines ranging from the 0.4th centile up to the 99.6th centile. The lines are taken from a large population of healthy children and show the wide variations in height and weight that are normal. (This information was collected in 1990 and is referred to as the 1990 Reference Chart for Age and Sex.) The 50th centile line represents the national average for white British children, with half of them falling above this line and the other half below. In order to see if the population today is getting heavier, the current average weight must be compared with the average from a previous time, for which the 1990 reference chart is used, or centile charts would be misleading. There are slightly different trends for children of other races, with Asian babies tending to be lighter and shorter and African-Caribbean babies tending to be heavier and longer on average. Examples of centile charts are found in Appendix 1.

The important thing about centile charts is that they predict how most people are likely to grow. If a baby's early measurements have followed the 75th centile

Table 3.1 Adult body mass index guide. (This does not apply under age 18)

BMI under 18.5	BMI between 18.5 and 24.9	BMI between 25 and 29.9	BMI between 30 and 39.9	BMI over 40
Underweight	Normal weight	Overweight	Obese	Morbidly obese*

* Morbid obesity means that there is a very high chance of developing weight-related illnesses, especially diabetes.

for weight then, by and large, they would be expected to follow that line during later childhood. Small changes are not unusual, such as dropping from the 75th to the 50th centile, but big changes, such as starting on the 25th and ending up on the 90th, require looking into.

What is body mass index?

Growth charts alone are not sufficient for showing if a person is either obese or underweight. A child may be on the 95th centile for weight but this does not necessarily mean they are overweight. If that child's height is also following the 95th centile then they may be just the right build, only taller than other children of the same age. In the same way, a child whose height and weight both fall on the 3rd centile may be petite but perfectly healthy, rather than underweight.

The height and weight measurements must be combined to see if a weight problem is present. This is done by using the body mass index, or BMI. The BMI gives a good (but not perfect) idea of whether a person is carrying too much body fat.

$$\text{BMI} = \frac{\text{weight (in kilograms)}}{\text{height squared (in metres)}}$$

For adults, BMI provides a simple guide to whether weight matches height appropriately, as outlined in Table 3.1.

For children, the BMI is more complex because it varies from birth to adulthood and is different between boys and girls. But it is still useful when plotted on a chart for comparison against the appropriate expected range. If a child's height and weight seem to be following different centile lines then it may be useful to calculate the BMI to check things further. Body mass index charts for boys and girls are given in Appendix 1. An online calculator for working out and interpreting a child's BMI is available at: www.healthforallchildren.co.uk on the parent's page.

Monitoring growth when measurements are not available

If there are no weight or height measurements available, a parent can still gain a rough idea about their child's growth by looking at other aspects:

• Clothes size. Whilst there is enormous variation in both children and in clothing manufacturers' sizing of children's clothes, they can still give an idea about whether a child is near the average or way off. If a young child always requires clothing that is designed for much older children then the chances are they are overweight. It is harder to tell if a child is underweight from clothing sizes because many skinny but healthy people will find that any trousers that fit the legs always have far too baggy a waistband.

- Compare with friends of the same age. Once again, with such huge variations in healthy growth patterns, it may not be helpful to compare one child next to another. However, if a child physically stands out from all the other children in their class at school then it may be a good idea to monitor height and weight more accurately to see if this is highlighting a problem.
- Teasing from other children. Sadly, tact is not usually a strong point of children and they will tell other children if they seem different to themselves. Teasing about weight or height from other children is very common and can lead to loss of confidence and unhappiness at school, and reluctance to take part in physical education (PE) or swimming. If a child has started to feel self-conscious and worried about their appearance then this might signal teasing due to weight, in which case it is time to check things out further.
- Family trends. If family members tend to be on the large size then the same tendency may apply to children of the household too. It is very common for children of overweight parents to become overweight themselves, so parents should give some thought to their child's build if they are overweight.
- Worrying signs. Children do not need to store rolls of fat even if they are shortly to start a growth spurt. Watch out for signs of a 'spare tyre' around the midriff or a tummy that hangs over the waistband, jowls or a double chin that hides the shape of the jaw, or pronounced fat across the chest giving the appearance of breasts in boys or in girls before the onset of puberty. The ribs should normally be visible in children as they raise and lower their arms.

How much exercise is a child getting?

Some parents know how active their child is without even having to think about it. The clues may be the holes in every item of their clothing, the fact that clean knees would be a noteworthy event or frequent despair from the window repair bill from stray footballs. Another group of parents will be fully aware of the opposite – that their children hate all exercise and the only hurrying they do is to find a seat. But many parents may be unsure: perhaps their children do some sports on occasion but exercise opportunities are limited. The Child Activity Assessment questions in Box 3.1 will help parents find out if their children are getting enough exercise for good health.

Box 3.1 Child Activity Assessment questions
- Is total television viewing less than 3.5 hours each day?
- Are there opportunities to play outside most days?
- Do the family get some exercise together, such as swimming, cycling or walking?
- Are the children able to walk to school?
- What about sports clubs or activity groups outside of school?

Reproduced from *Get Kids on the Go* by kind permission of the British Heart Foundation, 2004.

If the answers are all yes then that is a great start. If the answers are all no, then the children are almost certainly not getting enough exercise to keep healthy. If the answers are a mixture of yes and no, then it will be helpful to explore more opportunities for exercise. Aim for up to an hour of active play or sports, in addition to school PE, on most days of the week. Simply limiting time in front of the television has been shown to improve health, regardless of what a child does instead, although time spent playing computer games counts the same as watching TV.

Children will be active if they want to

Whether children choose to be active will be influenced by similar factors to those guiding their food choices. So children will:

- copy the activity patterns of parents and other role models
- play games that they have previously enjoyed and that are part of their familiar routine
- play games that wind up their parents, because that is fun
- do exercise that they *sense* is good for them or feels like a challenge, rather than because they've been *told* it is good for them
- do activities that are straightforward rather than require a lot of organising
- do things that appeal even if they've been told it's not a good idea.

For children who are enthusiastic about exercise but still seem to do little, it will help to assess the practical barriers that are stopping them. For children who hate exercise and find any excuse to stay indoors, the first task is to look at ways to improve motivation and interest in becoming more active, because opportunities will not be taken up unless they are appealing. Both these areas are covered in more detail in Chapters 7 and 11, but some of the principles are outlined here.

Practical barriers to being active

Previous generations of children were simply thrown outdoors to entertain themselves, but this has become less usual, particularly for younger children, because of our heightened awareness of safety. Most parents now feel they should know not only where their children are, but whom they are with and what conditions they are playing in. If parents are to personally supervise children then they need time to do it, but with far more parents out at work nowadays, parental time is also more pressured. These reasons mean it is easier to supervise at home, with children no longer encouraged to roam the district on their own. Children get bored easily indoors, and so television viewing and computer use increases.

A child's baseline activity can be increased by simple measures. Just being aware of how much television a child watches, and making efforts to reduce this, will have a beneficial effect. Make sure a child knows why limits are being introduced, and offer some suggestions for alternative activities, in order that it will be seen as a positive change.

If parents organise routines to include some simple extras, such as stopping off at a park, joining in with ball games or making time to walk to places instead of using the car, they will show their children that activity is important because they are taking the trouble to prioritise it. Seeing a parent take part in a sport is the best role model. After-school clubs are a good option for some children. What is available locally? If transport and pick-up times are barriers to this, it may be possible to team up with other parents.

If a child tried one activity but was put off in some way, do not be afraid to try another. For younger children, in particular, it is useful to plan several trials of different sports or activities, perhaps with coaching at a local sports hall, so that they can try out a few options as well as develop baseline skills in several different areas.

Make sure children have some basic sports equipment at home, such as footballs, rackets, skipping ropes or a skateboard, plus decent trainers, and take equipment along when out and about, in order to make the most of any opportunities to play.

How may a reluctant child be motivated?

We can't expect all kids to love football or swimming. Thankfully, being active doesn't have to mean wearing a sports kit or joining a team. Encourage children to look into a wide variety of activities, remembering that almost anything is better than watching television. What is more, making a small change over a long period is much better than a mammoth effort that doesn't continue for long. Little things can make a big difference, as long as they become a regular part of life.

An important part of motivating a child is to make health and fitness relevant, worthwhile and, above all, achievable so that current barriers are worth overcoming. This involves showing a child that all sorts of activities besides sports can help with fitness, and that worthwhile improvements can happen without necessarily having to join a team or get out of breath. For example, if a child loves charging round in the playground before school starts, but slows up over the rest of the day, then arriving five minutes early each day will mean 25 minutes' extra activity every week, for very little effort. Or if a child is in the habit of turning the television on as soon as they arrive home from school, suggest that it is not switched on for the first half an hour and that this is an unwinding time – time for some stretching and running about after a hard day's work. This may help break the habit of watching as much television because it allows the child to get on with other activities first, before the television has chance to grab the child's interest.

Look at the things a child currently enjoys to see if there are activity opportunities that might be linked. For example, if a girl loves Brownies then see if she can be encouraged to go for some of the more energetic badges. Be sure to capitalise on anything that a child is good at, as this will build confidence.

Household chores can, with a little thought, be modified to encourage activity (rather than the usual aim of making household chores as little trouble as possible). But for this to be successful, make sure they apply to everyone in the house. For example, do not leave things on the stairs – take them up and put them away. Avoid one journey carrying 'the lazy man's load' and go instead for several journeys carrying 'the fit man's load'. Get children used to taking some responsibility in the house from an early age, such as laying the table or taking the bin bag out, to help them feel like a valued member of the family team. A sense of self-worth is crucial in building self-confidence. Children won't object to sharing the work of a team that they feel they belong to, but they will object if they feel they are being asked to do the dirty jobs that everyone else hates. This problem can be avoided by making sure that everyone in the family takes turns with chores.

Sometimes it is a child's lack of self-confidence that is the main reason behind a dislike of exercise. Self-confidence can be bolstered in many ways, and is discussed in depth in later chapters, but a good starter is to make sure a child has mastered basic skills such as kicking a football, catching a ball and swimming.

Sometimes a history of illness or an ongoing condition such as asthma or a physical disability may interfere with both a child's ability to exercise and confidence in taking part. Specific conditions and illnesses are discussed in Chapter 15.

Summary points

- Children must want to exercise in order to do so out of choice.
- Children need to have opportunities to be active, both in terms of time and equipment.
- Children who lack motivation to exercise can be inspired to become more active.
- Self-confidence is crucial for children to join in.

Section 2

Pre-school children

From birth to around five years of age, children learn a huge amount about what foods they like and about normal family eating patterns. This section shows how to help pre-school children develop a taste for healthy foods so they will enjoy a varied diet, and how to avoid common behaviour problems that relate to meals.

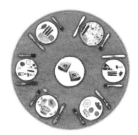

Chapter 4

Milk, weaning and promoting healthy foods

Breast or bottle – does it matter?

It is one of the most personal of choices, whether to breast or bottle-feed a baby, and only a mother will know how she feels about it. We are fortunate to have very safe and nutritionally suitable formula milk for mothers who do not wish to breast-feed or who have been unable to get breast-feeding established, but formula milk is not as complete as breast milk in providing everything a baby needs.

Wherever possible, give breast-feeding a try and see how things go: many women find it is worth a bit of effort in the early weeks because of the many benefits once it is well established (*see* Box 4.1). Roughly 65% of UK women try breast-feeding, with around 40% still doing so by the time their baby is six weeks old.

Box 4.1 The benefits of breast-feeding

- Breast milk contains antibodies, which give extra protection from infection in the months before a baby's own immune system becomes effective.
- Breast milk can alter in strength and quality to fit the needs of a baby according to things like illness or hot weather.
- Breast milk is very convenient, requiring no preparation or sterilising, and is usually provided in the exact quantity that a baby demands. Night-time feeds in particular are simple.
- Breast milk is cheap – a new mother merely needs to eat a reasonably balanced diet herself in order to produce it.
- Unlike formula milk, there is no need to keep breast milk cool when out and about – it is available at the right temperature when required.
- Breast-feeding helps the womb to return more quickly to its normal size after childbirth.
- A breast-feeding mother will use up some of the fat stores that were laid down during pregnancy, helping her to regain her pre-pregnancy weight more easily.
- Once breast-feeding is fully established, milk can be expressed and either kept in a fridge or frozen (using sterile equipment), so that a mother can go out without her baby.

For those mums who are not able to breast-feed or who choose not to try, formula milk will provide the correct balance of nutrition for a new baby and has the added benefit that feeding can be shared with baby's father or other family or friends.

Formula milk is produced from specially modified cow's milk, which is altered so that babies can digest it easily and so that it has the correct balance of vitamins and minerals. Ordinary cow's milk, goat's milk, condensed, evaporated or dried milk should not be used at all for babies until over a year old.

If a mother is HIV-positive she will be advised not to breast-feed because the virus can be passed through breast milk to her baby. Some drugs and alcohol can also pass into breast milk, so keep alcohol to a bare minimum and check with a doctor about any drugs that are prescribed when breast-feeding.

Getting breast-feeding established

For such a natural activity, it is surprising that breast-feeding generates such a degree of debate. In some western countries, including the UK, there is still a slightly prudish attitude that makes some women feel either embarrassed or uncomfortable about breast-feeding in public. This is a pity because it adds a little more pressure at a time when women typically feel unsure of themselves.

It is important for women to feel good about breast-feeding because it can take some determination to get through the first few weeks. Whilst some women take to breast-feeding easily, most women find the first few weeks uncomfortable or sometimes even painful, whilst the nipples get used to regular feeds. Even though discomfort can be reduced by carefully helping the baby to latch on and by making sure that there is a comfortable chair with good back support, many women find the first two weeks hard work. However, it improves dramatically once milk flow becomes established and the new baby has got the hang of what to do, enabling mum to become more confident in the whole process.

Having good support is a bonus, so midwife support is usually available in the early weeks. Health visitors help with breast-feeding after midwife input has stopped. Ask relatives, friends and neighbours for advice, too, if they had positive experiences of breast-feeding themselves. The National Childbirth Trust and the La Leche League can also give support through other mothers who have experience of breast-feeding (*see* Appendix 2 for details).

Tips for successful breast-feeding

Anxiety is very common amongst almost all new mothers. Advice about how to look after new babies is rife, with even passers-by in the street likely to offer an opinion. The first few weeks of breast-feeding – when a baby may lose weight rather than gain it and when a mother feels sore and tired – are bound to have their ups and downs. The following section aims to boost confidence in getting breast-feeding established.

- Ignore any advice that causes confusion or worry: every woman has her own inbuilt baby-care manual called 'the maternal instinct'. Tuning in to this at an early stage will allow each mother to bring up her own baby in the way that she wants.

- If not sure what to do then do seek advice – but bear in mind the point above! Midwives, health visitors and some family doctors and practice nurses may all be able to answer queries or give a little more support, in addition to family and friends. Sometimes mothers are given conflicting advice from different people – in that case, choose the advice that makes most sense or do your own thing altogether.
- Understand about milk flow. Surprisingly, babies do not have a huge appetite in the first few days after being born. Of course they need some nourishment, but to begin with breast milk is thick and highly concentrated (this is called colostrum). It is full of antibodies to help fight infection plus some nourishment. Babies do not need much in order to get by.
- After being squeezed and squashed through the very tight birth canal, many newborn babies have a bit of a headache and may feel exhausted. This can mean that a baby is not interested in feeding much for the first 12 to 24 hours. If a baby is healthy in every other way, then be guided by their interest in feeding. They will undoubtedly be more awake by day two, but if there is undue sleepiness then ask for advice at this stage.
- New mums can feel utterly exhausted after childbirth because of the effort and adrenaline rush involved, making the emotional strain of trying to breast-feed straight away rather daunting. Taking time and beginning with short feeds is fine because the colostrum is so thick and rich that only small quantities are needed in the first few days.
- If a baby seems to suckle for hours on end, he or she is doing so only for comfort. Almost all of the milk or colostrum will be taken during the first 10 to 15 minutes, making long feeds unnecessary – unless both mother and baby are happy to continue for longer.
- Milk arrives in dramatic fashion on about day four. The sudden arrival of hugely engorged breasts may come as a shock or feel as though a pair of footballs have become attached to the chest! Now that there is some milk to drink, a baby may find they get a face-full before even managing to latch on, because the let-down reflex (the tingling sensation that means milk is being released into the milk ducts) can mean that milk spurts forth. The other breast may leak during a feed, so some women use 'breast shells' to collect the extra milk if breast pads are not absorbent enough. Milk supply settles down into a more predictable supply over the first four weeks or so, as routines start to develop.
- If a new mum finds the first couple of days very stressful and feels like giving up, there is no reason why she shouldn't have another go once her milk comes in, on around day four. Milk supply will build up according to how often the baby suckles so breast-feeding can re-establish even if there has been a lapse of a day or two. If she has stopped for longer than a couple of days then it will be harder for breast-feeding to re-establish properly.
- If breast-feeding is causing worry and distress, then be happy that giving colostrum in the first four to five days is a fantastic start because of the extra protection against infection that the baby receives. Persevering to day five is really good, but the longer the better. Babies should, if possible, be exclusively breast-fed until around six months old.
- If a new mum is having a really bad day, then it is not the end of the world to resort to a bottle. If she is keen to keep trying with breast-feeding, a one-off

bottle-feed will not ruin all chances of breast-feeding again, and it may take the pressure off for a few hours. It is preferable to breast-feed exclusively where possible, but it is better for a mum to feel she is coping (even if that means an occasional bottle-feed) than for her to become exhausted, with cracked nipples and to feel like a failure.

- It is normal and expected for newborn babies to lose weight in the first week and to regain birth weight by the end of the first two weeks. Bottle-fed babies are less likely to lose as much weight, but this does not give a bottle-fed baby any advantage over a breast-fed one because things even out in the end. This is not a reflection of breast milk not being up to the job, it is the way nature is designed. It is more important for a newborn baby to stock up with immune protection against infection than to start an early growth spurt.

- If a new baby is crying, the solution is not always milk. If a new mum always offers a feed whenever her baby cries, this can be a cause of painful nipples. If a baby has been fed within the last hour and a half, then try something else to settle them before offering another feed. Going for a walk in the pushchair, having a nappy change or a bath, or simply being handed to a different member of the family are all options to try for a well-fed but crying baby.

- Well-meaning relatives and friends can sometimes say the wrong thing. If any kindly souls are busy suggesting that a new mum could do things differently then either hand them the ironing and tell them to keep quiet or suggest they call again in a few weeks' time! It is normal for new mums to go through a very sensitive phase.

- New breast-feeding mums should be forbidden from making the tea for calling visitors. If visitors are looking thirsty then a quick explanation of where the tea things are should give them the hint. Experienced mums having a third or fourth baby are more likely to explain to their visitors where the vacuum cleaner is, rather than the tea things!

How much milk is enough?

Regardless of whether a baby is breast- or bottle-fed, you can remain confident about whether a baby is taking enough milk by remembering the following:

- Rely on a baby's growth rather than milk intake or time taken to feed when assessing progress. If a baby seems to take very little but is growing beautifully, then there is little to worry about. Some babies become very efficient at taking in all they need in a very short time, whereas other babies like to take their time when feeding.

- There is no need to measure and monitor how much milk a baby drinks in normal circumstances. If there is illness with sickness and diarrhoea, then it may be helpful to note the frequency of feeds and, more importantly, how often the baby has a wet nappy. It is less important to know how much formula has been taken – a breast-feeding mother will not know anyway. A doctor will be able to tell if a baby has enough fluid on board or whether there are signs of dehydration by examining the baby and asking about the number of wet nappies that day.

- If a mother feels she wants to monitor the amount of milk a baby drinks, she should assess milk intake over 24-hour periods, rather than individual feeds, which can vary throughout the day.
- It is not a concern if one small feed is quickly followed by a demand for another. A baby will get used to how much is really wanted with a bit of practice.
- Try not to object to demands for extra feeds during hot weather, even if a baby was previously in a nice routine. Things will soon settle back to normal once the stress of hot weather is over.
- Be aware of growth spurts and how this can affect a baby's milk requirements. During active growth, a baby will increase either the amount of milk taken during a feed or the number of feeds each day. But following a growth spurt they may take less milk again for a while, rather than sticking to the increased amount.
- Where possible, try to breast-feed.

The weaning process

At around 4–6 months a baby will be weaned onto pureed foods, which gradually get lumpier as the months progress and teeth arrive to help with chewing. There is no good reason to start this process too soon, although many mothers sense pressure from relatives and friends to introduce solids early on. Ignore them! If a baby is getting hungrier at around four months of age then increase the frequency of milk feeds: more milk more often will do the trick.

The World Health Organization guidelines currently recommend that, wherever possible, all babies should be exclusively breast-fed up to six months of age. An approved formula milk is a suitable alternative if breast-feeding is not possible.

I did not manage to achieve this with any of my three children, and felt a lot of pressure to introduce solids from around 12 weeks of age. I managed to hold out to 16 weeks before introducing a little baby rice. Because all three of my babies loved solids and wolfed down any that were offered, I understand how families tend to feel that solids are a good thing and that earlier introduction might be best.

There are, however, very good reasons for delaying things until at least four months of age or six months if possible:

- Milk is the best food for the early months when a baby's brain and other organs are growing rapidly and the immune system is still immature. Breast milk provides immune protection, reducing the chance of infections – in particular, diarrhoea and sickness bugs. Even though formula milk does not contain a mother's antibodies, like breast milk does, at least it can be prepared in a sterile way, but it is far harder to sterilise solids. As a baby grows and their immune system works more effectively, the need for everything to be sterile becomes less important.
- Babies have to learn how to swallow solids, as they are trickier to swallow than milk. Introducing them before a baby is ready increases the chance of choking, which can lead to coughs and upper respiratory infections. Even if a young baby seems keen to try solids, the swallowing mechanism will be

immature, which may explain why babies that are weaned early (under four months) are more likely to have infections of the upper airways throughout their first year.

- Introducing certain foods too soon can result in allergies. Peanuts should not be given to babies or children under the age of two because of the risk of choking. (Peanuts can cause a nasty lung reaction if they go down the wrong way and enter the lungs.) But even pureed peanut should be avoided because of the chance of developing peanut allergy (*see* Chapter 15 for more details on peanut and other food allergies).

- Wheat and other gluten-containing foods should be avoided until over six months of age. This is due to the small risk of developing coeliac disease, a condition where the gut reacts to gluten in foods, causing diarrhoea, difficulties absorbing food and hence failure to thrive. Gluten is found in most cereals and flour, but rice, fruit and vegetables are naturally gluten-free. Commercial weaning foods are usually well labelled to show which products are suitable. Look for 'gluten-free' on the packaging up to the age of six months. After this age, wheat and other cereals can be safely introduced. However, if there is a family history of coeliac disease then this should be discussed with a doctor to decide on the best time to introduce gluten into the baby's diet. Late weaning is probably a good idea for any baby that is considered a high risk for allergies.

Most mothers start weaning with either pureed vegetables, baby rice or gluten-free rusk mixed with the baby's usual milk. Start towards the end of a milk feed when baby is no longer hungry, then gradually build up the amount offered at that mealtime before adding small amounts of solids at different times of the day. Other purees are gradually added such as vegetable, potato, pulse or fruit purees, plus dairy products such as yoghurts and custard. Later, as small lumps are tolerated, it is time to add proteins such as cheese, minced meat and fish. If any food is refused, try it again another day until the baby gradually gets used to all the usual foods that are going to be on offer. Babies take time to get used to new textures and flavours.

Finger foods help to develop co-ordination and a sense of independence, whilst encouraging chewing practice.

What about milk during the weaning process?

Milk remains the most important ingredient of a baby's diet until at least a year old, because it contains essential protein, calcium and vitamins as well as being a good source of energy. Breast-feeding, if going well, can be continued happily and, if a mother is able to express extra milk, it can be mixed in with weaning foods to help with accepting new flavours.

Expressed milk can be kept fresh in a sterile container in the fridge for 24 hours, or can be frozen in small sterile bags and used as required. Hand or battery pumps are widely available, and some maternity units have expressing pumps available to borrow. Make sure the equipment is scrupulously sterilised according to the instructions before each use.

Do not be surprised at the appearance of breast milk when it has been left standing. It is high in fat and this separates out, giving a thick fatty layer on top and much more watery milk underneath. Stirring or shaking it will quickly combine the two layers.

Pasteurised cow's milk can be used to make up weaning foods but should not be given as the usual drink until over one year. Its low levels of vitamin D and iron make it unsuitable for the mainstay of an infant's diet. Also, because cow's milk is more energy-dense than human milk, giving it to young babies can lead to dehydration, because the baby will fill up on calories before taking in enough fluid. Semi-skimmed milk can be used for children over two years if they are eating well and getting plenty of energy from the rest of their diet. Fully skimmed milk, however, should not be given as a main drink until aged five at least because it is low in both calories and vitamins.

The benefits of weaning

Not only is weaning great fun, but it is a vital part of a baby's development. Many families will have charming photographs of their baby splattered from head to toe in mush, or snapshots of the funny faces babies pull as they experience a new flavour. They are images to treasure! But weaning is a vital step for a number of reasons:

- Firstly, whilst milk is ideal up to six months of age, it won't suffice alone forever. Breast milk is low in minerals such as iron and vitamins A and D (although they are added to formula milk). By about six months the stores a baby has at birth will be running low, so this is the time to add in other foods to get the balance back.
- Babies need lots of energy, and protein in particular, to keep pace with their rapid growth. Moving on to solids will help them get the increasing calories they need without having a tummy sloshing with milk.
- A baby must develop strength of the mouth muscles in order to eat solids, which is also excellent preparation for learning to talk because this uses the same muscles.

Weaning can be a great time to take the pressure off mum and allow dad or other family to get involved with feeding the baby. It is a time for babies to discover that they belong to a family and to start copying what everyone else does at the table.

Weaning guidelines

Whilst the aim of weaning is to gradually teach children to eat anything that might be on offer, there are a few starting guidelines that help with safety. By the age of one, a baby should be eating solids several times a day, and be joining in with family meals. Full progress onto the family's complete variety of foods will depend on chewing ability, which depends on when the back (molar) teeth erupt.

- Young children should always be supervised at mealtimes. Watch for signs of choking as well as making sure that an infant can't slide out of the high chair.
- Sugar and salt should not be added to infant foods. A young baby's kidneys are not designed to deal with lots of salt, and giving salt to a young baby can cause

dehydration. If a child learns to like eating salty foods (because they are served often), it will increase the risk of developing high blood pressure later in life. Weaning on to very sugary foods will encourage a 'sweet tooth', and may lead to the baby rejecting blander basic foods. Added salt and sugar should be reserved until the baby is over a year, and then used sparingly.

- Children should eat something from the following groups each day and so the weaning process should gradually introduce foods from each group so that they become familiar:
  - cereal foods and starchy vegetables, such as breads, potatoes and rice
  - fruit and vegetables
  - protein foods, e.g. meat, fish, eggs, pulses and beans. There is no need to go for low-fat foods in young babies; full-fat dairy products are suitable.
- Avoid heavily spiced foods. Let children get used to mild tastes and new textures before bombarding the taste buds with spices. Adding delicate flavours with a few herbs is a good start before progressing onto stronger flavours as weaning becomes well established.
- Avoid all nuts and other foods that are associated with allergy, such as shellfish and prawns. See Chapter 15 for more details on peanut allergy and other food intolerances.
- Ensure eggs are thoroughly cooked or hard-boiled in order to avoid salmonella, which can cause food poisoning.
- Leave pâté and those smelly soft cheeses (known as mould-ripened soft cheeses), such as Brie, until a child is older. These foods can be associated with Listeria, an infection that can cause a serious flu-like illness in young babies. It is also dangerous in pregnancy as it can be associated with miscarriage and stillbirth. In healthy children and adults the immune system will fight this infection without a problem, so these foods are safe after the first two years.
- Teach a child early on to get used to drinking from a beaker or cup. Milk can still be given in a bottle if preferred, but giving juice or other drinks through a teat is strongly associated with tooth decay. Vary the drinks offered and make sure that water is offered several times each day, especially between meals.
- Limit high-fibre foods until a child is over a year. They do not need to be avoided completely, but babies cannot cope with too much fibre in their gut and it can cause frequent loose motions. Some wholegrain breakfast cereals (like Weetabix), whilst mashing to a nice consistency that most babies like, can be a cause of baby diarrhoea. However, some babies are prone to very hard motions, in which case increasing fibre in the diet is the healthiest way to improve things and a wholegrain breakfast cereal may be suitable. A parent may need to experiment to find what is most suitable.
- Iron-rich foods should be incorporated into a baby's diet. Iron is needed to help carry oxygen in the blood and a shortage can lead to anaemia. Vitamin C helps the body to absorb iron, so combine foods so that a meal provides both of these ingredients (*see* Box 4.2). There has been concern about how common anaemia is in young children, with around 9% of young children having iron stores low enough to lead to anaemia.

Box 4.2 Foods rich in iron and vitamin C

Foods rich in iron

- Red meat: beef, pork, lamb
- Poultry
- Liver and liver sausage
- Oily fish
- Fish fingers
- Eggs
- Green leafy vegetables
- Beans and lentils
- Breakfast cereal with added iron
- Baby foods with added iron
- Dried fruits, e.g. apricots

Foods rich in vitamin C

- Citrus fruits, e.g. oranges
- Unsweetened fruit juice (serve diluted)
- Summer fruits, e.g. peaches, strawberries
- Green leafy vegetables
- Tomatoes, green pepper, peas
- Potatoes

Should babies and young children be given vitamin supplements?

In the UK, the Department of Health currently recommends that children from one to five years of age should receive routine supplementation of vitamins A, C and D. For breast-fed babies this should start at six months of age (although this should be considered from one month of age if the mother has had problems with nutrition herself during the pregnancy). Bottle-fed babies receive vitamins A and D in their formula or follow-on milk, and so do not need to start supplements until one year of age.

Overdosing on vitamins A or D can be harmful, so do not be tempted to double up on doses 'for good measure'.

Oral drops are available free of charge to families receiving Income Support or an income-based Jobseeker's Allowance. Otherwise they are available direct to the public from maternity and child health clinics.

Vitamin deficiency illnesses are rare in the UK and will be even more unlikely if a baby is gradually weaned onto a well-balanced diet that contains the recommended minimum five portions of fruit and vegetables each day. Details of portion sizes for fruit and vegetables for young children are given in Chapter 12.

Advice for premature babies may be different from the above, so you will need to consult a doctor or maternity unit for more information.

Summary points

- Breast-feeding is undoubtedly best, but bottle-feeding has merits too. It takes commitment in order to get breast-feeding established in the early weeks, but there is plenty of help available for those mums who find it difficult.
- Always let a baby decide on how much milk is taken, rather than forcing them to take more than is wanted. It usually takes four or more weeks for a feeding pattern to begin to establish, during which time 'demand feeding' is the best approach.
- Weaning should be a slow process because there is such a lot for babies to learn. Milk remains very important throughout the first year and beyond, regardless of how popular solids are.
- The weaning process should introduce as many varied foods and flavours as possible to help establish a balanced diet. This will ensure that there are plenty of vitamins, minerals and fibre for good growth, without the problems of too much sugar and salt.

Chapter 5

Developing a taste for the healthy things in life

This chapter looks at the opportunities for introducing young children to the healthy things in life and explains the Four P's approach to making these seem worth a try. Food is ranked according to how special it is, which provides an opening for making ordinary things a little more exciting and hence more popular. Putting healthy foods in reach can make a big difference to whether young children choose them.

The 'food window'

Milk is the only thing on offer for roughly the first four months of a baby's life. Rather than finding this boring, babies demand their milk as if their lives depend on it – which of course is the case. It is when solids are introduced that the problems usually begin.

Tolerating a varied diet does not necessarily come easily. How can a young baby be taught to move from that easy-to-swallow, sweet, warm, totally satisfying drink onto lumps that may be hard, spicy, hot, cold, salty, gooey or dry? In a nutshell, babies learn slowly, by trying new foods again and again until they become familiar, and, at the same time, continuing to drink plenty of milk to supply enough energy during this process. It doesn't matter that babies learn slowly, because childhood lasts a long time, so as long as new foods keep reappearing they will eventually become familiar and a baby will begin to like them.

From about the age of eight months to just over a year, babies have a sort of 'food window' – a time when they will tolerate just about anything that is on offer. Not the first time, and perhaps not the second either, but in general, during this phase of development, the more varied foods a baby tries, the more likely they will cope with a varied diet later on. Babies get used to the idea of not knowing what might come next, but a baby weaned onto only a few bland foods at this time may struggle to enjoy strange textures and flavours later on, giving the impression of a fussy eater.

Variety – why bother?

There are many reasons why a varied diet is important. Here are some of them:

- Lots of different nutrients are needed to create a balanced diet but most foods contain some rather than all of the essential items. Eating a variety of foods from each of the food groups, as described in *The Balance of Good Health* (*see*

Chapter 1), will give the full range of essentials without worrying about specific ingredients because eating a bit of this and a bit of that will cover all the basics. A limited diet is far more likely to be short of at least some of the essential nutrients. One example is iron, which is found in meat and fish, cereals and some green vegetables. Up to 9% of teenage girls are low in iron stores, putting them at risk of anaemia as they continue to develop.

- Children who eat a varied diet are easier to feed, especially when away from home when normal food items are not available, such as when visiting friends or eating in restaurants.
- Children who eat a varied diet will gain interest from their food as they explore new textures, flavours and food combinations.
- Children who do not mind eating whatever is put in front of them will not mind if parents decide to go on a health drive. If a family decides that fried foods should be kept for occasional treats and to go for jacket potatoes and pasta instead, children will follow suit with little fuss.
- A child who enjoys a varied diet that includes lots of fruit and vegetables will eat proportionately less high-fat or high-sugar foods, thus reducing the chance of being overweight or obese.

Balancing pushing new flavours with allowing children a choice

Chapters 1 and 2 looked at how important it is for children to be able to make their own choices about food, particularly the quantity of food eaten. This allows them to tune in to what their own appetite is telling them, rather than feeling obliged to clear their plate. However, this doesn't fit well with very young children, who may be reluctant to try new foods at all if not encouraged to do so. Indeed many parents feel that it is an effort to get young children to eat anything, let alone try new foods. It can be reassuringly tempting to offer tried and tested bland or sugary foods that will get eaten, rather than offer new items that may end up in the bin. Remember that a balanced diet is important and will be worth a bit of effort (*see* Box 5.1).

Box 5.1 Tips for successful introduction of new foods during the weaning process

Parents should be prepared to:

- throw food away
- offer tiny amounts of new things – a large portion of anything can look rather threatening
- offer new foods in different settings, such as for snacks, when out and about, and when a child is bored
- join in by eating the new food too
- keep offering the new food from time to time regardless of a child's initial reaction
- serve the new food in different ways, such as boiled, raw, mashed or mixed with other ingredients

- offer two new foods at a time, so that one of them might seem nicer than the other. This gives a child a sense of choice over what is on offer, even though both foods are new.

The Four P's approach to helping children eat healthily

Having already established that in order for children to eat fruit and vegetables, or other healthy things, they must be enjoyable, the challenge for parents is to help children develop a taste for the healthy things in life, so that there is no need for any coaxing into unwilling mouths. The Four P's approach can help pre-school children grow to like the foods that the family eats:

- Parental example – a vital part of how a child learns to accept new foods
- Packaging – making foods appear attractive
- Persuasion – using games and gimmicks to interest children in the food
- Persistence – continuing to quietly offer a food as many as ten times, whatever the first reaction to it, until it becomes familiar and acceptable.

Parental example

For this age group, a parent's example is very important, in addition to factors such as packaging, presentation and other links that are made with food. It is vital that a young child sees parents and family members enjoying the foods that will be served often. Offering snippets of information about why particular ingredients are good for us (such as carrots help people to see in the dark) will help a child become interested and more familiar with them. Offering small mouthfuls of 'grown-up' food from a parent's plate can make a food seem more intriguing, because children like to investigate things that they think are not allowed.

Packaging

Supermarkets are now full of foods aimed at young children, but many of these foods are high in sugar and salt. Yoghurts, biscuits, cereals, crisps and battered bits (such as nuggets) are often linked to film characters or TV shows, or have free toys or special offers that make the food item more appealing to young children. This tactic works well, but instead of helping children get hooked on junk food, the food industry's same principles can be used to promote healthier foods at home (*see* Box 5.2).

Box 5.2 Ideas for 'home marketing' of healthy foods

- Put sliced fruit or vegetables in a pot with a favourite cartoon picture on it to make the food seem a little more enticing than if it were presented whole or on a plain plate. Perhaps try eggcups or leftover party plates.
- Mix healthy snack ingredients with less healthy ones to improve the overall balance of the snack and to encourage the healthy ingredients to be eaten, e.g. add a few chocolate chips to a pot of raisins or chopped

fruit, or sprinkle moist apple segments with a few hundreds and thousands. Try a fondue, with lots of pieces of chopped fruit to dip into a little melted chocolate or sauce designed for ice-cream.

- Decorate some plain paper plates to create home-made gimmicky table-ware.
- Put healthy snacks in (clean) toy vehicles or on the doll's house kitchen table.
- Food that is eaten in the play tent, at a grandparents' house or on special occasions such as birthdays may appear more special than ordinary meals in the kitchen.
- Food can be fun as well as tasty. Turn apple or orange segments into miniature boats, or cut out pieces of apple into mini vehicles for small toy people or animals. Just making a small gouge in the side of a carrot can turn it – with a child's imaginative eye – into a submarine, a torpedo, a huge nose or whatever a child fancies.

Persuasion and mealtime games

Mealtime games are both fun and useful as they can encourage a child to eat. For young children they are especially useful for introducing new foods and flavours. Games such as 'Here comes the train into the tunnel' (i.e. mouth) can keep a child eating happily for as long as the game seems fun. But be clear about what a child is learning from mealtime games. In the early days they help to make strange new foods seem worth a try, but be cautious about using the same game to override a child's natural appetite and help them clear the plate, because recognising fullness is such an important aspect of eating sensibly in the long run.

An American study showed that up to the age of three, a child will eat what is wanted and leave the rest, but already by five years old will tend to clear a plateful of food even if portion sizes are made bigger than normal. This suggests that natural fullness cues can be overridden from this early age, putting children at increased risk of obesity in later years, and that the essential regulatory mechanism can be forgotten almost before it has had chance to begin.

Other studies have shown that young children regulate how much they eat over 24 hours, rather than at each mealtime. So a child who seems to eat next to nothing at mealtimes is likely to either snack later, fill up at a different meal that day or get sufficient nourishment from milk drinks. Worrying over poor intake at one meal is unnecessary. Monitor a child's general growth instead to see if the overall intake is adequate (*see* Chapter 3).

When a child is cajoled to eat 'one more mouthful' it introduces a new issue: the pleading on a parent's face and then the change to congratulatory joy after a mouthful disappears can teach children to eat simply to please a parent, rather than because of hunger. Indeed some children may go on to refuse everything unless a game is played, because of discovering such a reliable way to get attention. Broadening the way that games are played can weaken the link between mealtime attention and being fed. Children will quickly relearn that games can be enjoyed at any time if similar games are played in between meals too. Mealtime games are useful for introducing variety, but should not be used to force a child to overeat.

Persistence

There is a fine line between being invited to try something unfamiliar and being pressurised into trying something that is unwanted. If a parent is tense and concerned at mealtimes, worrying over whether things are tried or not, this can become a game in itself, with all sorts of food being rejected just to test out the parent's reaction. If a food keeps reappearing without any fuss or notice and the rest of the family seem to happily tuck in then young children are more likely to follow suit eventually, even though it may take many low-key appearances for this to happen.

Understand how food is ranked in a hierarchy

People learn to rank foods, whether consciously or subconsciously, according to how special they are. For example, bread is usually rated as just an ordinary, everyday food that varies in how nice it is depending on freshness and what is put on top of it. People do not usually give it much thought because it is such a basic part of the diet. However, chocolate-chip ice-cream with hot fudge sauce is a special food, not one for every day, and one that will usually generate a bit of discussion plus possible arguments about who had the largest portion and who will be allowed a second helping. Whilst it is being served a parent might comment on how expensive it was to buy, the trouble there was getting it home without it melting, or perhaps the family might remember a special occasion when this particular food was last eaten. It might be served in special fancy glasses, have a wafer stuck on the top, or be eaten with special sundae spoons. Any of these factors will create the impression that the food is special and worth coveting, regardless of how good it tastes. Children will register how highly the food was ranked by the amount of fuss it generated.

This doesn't mean that creating a big fuss over any food will automatically make it a favourite. The food itself must taste reasonably good or be so impressive to look at that it doesn't matter about the flavour.

Remembering that foods are rated according to how much interest and excitement they generate is very useful when introducing new healthy foods. It may only require one exciting 'food performance' for an everlasting impression to be made, such as using beetroot water for dyeing a T-shirt. Pineapple is another example. It has quite a strong flavour, an odd texture and an unusual smell, so many people might dislike it first time. However, by involving children in its preparation, allowing them to hold and smell it before it is peeled and sliced, then discovering the unusual fruit inside with its hard core is likely to make the fruit worthy of a try. The discarded leafy top can even be planted to see if it will grow. The next time pineapple is served, it could be chopped into different shapes whilst discussing whether the attempts to grow the leafy top worked or if it just went mouldy. Children will remember some of the intriguing business of eating fresh pineapple rather than whether they liked its flavour, so that it becomes an interesting food.

The aim when making a new food interesting is to generate an initial liking for it (*see* Box 5.3). It won't always be necessary to make a song and dance about the way it is served, because once the family have given it the thumbs-up the food should speak for itself. Equally, if despite the fascination factor the kids persist in spitting it out, then feel free to leave it off the shopping list.

Box 5.3 A few fascination factors

- Carrots: carefully nibble off the outside layer to leave the inner spiky stalk.
- Bananas: break in half then gently squeeze to divide into three length-ways portions.
- Avocados: the stone will sprout if it is supported in a jar of water. Roots will sprout from the bottom and then leaves will develop from the top. It can then be potted into some compost and be kept on a windowsill as a houseplant. Alternatively, slice lengthways and remove the stone to make excellent boats with a ready-made cabin to fill with either a bit of salad dressing, chopped-up bacon or whatever a child prefers. Or, if the avocado half is peeled, it can be sliced thinly then gently pushed sideways to create a beautiful fan.
- Beetroot: after boiling, use the water to dye an old T-shirt.
- Asparagus: this makes wee (urine) smell funny for a few hours.
- Sweet corn: this might appear in the loo the next day.
- Mangos: they make excellent hedgehogs. Slice in half with a sharp knife and remove the stone. Slice through the flesh in a crisscross pattern, taking care not to slice right through the outer skin (or your finger). Then gently turn inside out to reveal the hedgehog. Affix a cherry or a grape for his nose.
- Kiwis: eat with a teaspoon like a boiled egg.
- Mushrooms: these can be grown at home using a kit that is kept in the bathroom – no garden required. Ask at a local garden centre.
- Peas in the pod: ideal for perfecting counting skills and comparing if each pod contains the same number of peas.
- Sugar snap peas: offer them whole or open them for eating pea by pea.
- Parsnips: these make excellent crisps by slicing thinly and dry-roasting until crisp.
- Bean sprouts: purchase hard mung beans then put some in a shallow dish of water. They will sprout into bean sprouts after a few days, which can be eaten raw or thrown into a salad or stir-fry.
- Any home-grown food is likely to taste more interesting than something purchased in a shop.

Young children eat what they can reach

Parents have total control over the foods that a young child can reach. Toddlers strapped in pushchairs or car seats are a captive audience, which means they can only eat what is on offer. This creates a great opportunity for offering healthy foods in addition to crisps or sweets, because the overriding feeling when trapped in a pushchair is usually boredom rather than hunger. Anything that relieves boredom is likely to be appreciated regardless of how sugary or salty it is, so crunchy cucumber, a pot of fiddly raisins or a lump of cheese may all liven up dull moments. What is more, any food that has brought some relief to a dull day will seem more attractive in future, and so pushchair opportunities can boost the popularity of ordinary things. Variety is the key – sometimes crisps, sometimes fruit, sometimes a breadstick and occasionally sweets – because the more a child gets used to eating whatever arrives, the less likely there will be a tantrum if a specific item is unavailable. Make sure young children do not learn to associate a trip in the pushchair with a packet of crisps, because they won't always be to hand.

At home, if fruit is out of reach, it will get eaten less frequently than if it is on the table, put into grubby fingers, popped into chattering mouths and used to make the play food more interesting. Do not expect young children to ask for fruit; if it is handed out often enough, children will start to ask for it as they get a little older or will simply learn to help themselves.

Check with a child's nursery or child-minder that fruit and vegetables are offered several times a day. One slice of limp cucumber is not quite enough to keep the diet well balanced. Children who are reluctant to try healthy foods are more likely to do so if they see other children eating them, so if a child is struggling, child-care settings can encourage children to copy others who are good eaters.

Children will benefit from clear food rules

House rules are tremendously important in teaching children how to behave, so that they are ready to mix happily in the wider world as they grow. A child who is taught clear boundaries will find the world far less confusing than if the rules are constantly changing.

Different families have many unspoken rules that apply to food. A young child will gradually pick up all the family ways such as how everyone places their knife and fork at the end of a meal, asking to leave the table, swapping leftovers at the end of a meal, whether everyone grazes in front of the TV and any number of other habits that each family tends to follow.

Some house rules are worth changing because they may be ones that were simply remembered from childhood, rather than rules that are worth enforcing. An example might be the now out-of-date notion that children should be seen and not heard. Some rules are for safety ('do not put your knife in your mouth'), some are for hygiene or health reasons ('do not put your feet on the table' and 'wash your hands before eating'), but some are simply to make our lives easier ('will you please not throw food because I find it tedious to clear it up').

House rules can be introduced to help a child eat sensibly; for example, if hungry at the end of a meal then a child may help themselves to fruit or a piece of bread. Be aware of the tendency for children to test rules as they grow. If a rule is worthwhile then without making too big an issue, gently stick to it. But equally, if a rule is causing more trouble than it's worth, make a clear change, if necessary explaining to children why the change is being made. Rules are there to be useful and to simplify both life and the process of growing up, rather than to make life awkward and difficult. Avoid rules that force a child to eat things that are disliked, or that encourage eating after feeling full.

Young children copy their parents' eating patterns

This includes troublesome or quirky eating patterns. Many parents eat in odd ways or have strong emotions over food, which young children will pick up and look on as normal behaviour. This might include seeing parents eat wacky diets, noticing that grown-ups sometimes feel guilty after eating, that sneaking an extra treat is a way to cope with feeling sad and that if someone misses out on food the rest of the family are eating they feel hard done by. These issues are significant because they can pave the way for a child to develop eating problems later in life.

Parents should aim to provide good, wholesome food and insist on the family sitting down to eat together for as many meals as possible. Everyone should eat roughly the same food, even if quantities vary. There is good research to show that regular family meals (where the family sit down together) can result in healthier foods being eaten, with greater fruit and vegetable consumption and a greater likelihood of children eating breakfast the next day, which is always the best start to the day.

Summary points

- From about eight months of age, introduce as much variety as possible into a child's diet.
- Use food games and fascination factors to help a child develop a liking for healthy foods.
- Do not be tempted to use food games to override a child's natural appetite.
- Make the foods that children should eat easily accessible.
- Sort out parental eating problems if children are not to copy them.
- Encourage the family to eat together on a regular basis.

Chapter 6

Understanding problem eaters

Eating problems are very common and cause much parental anxiety and concern. However, growth is not always affected, and it can be monitored in order to see if an eating tendency is affecting growth. This chapter looks at what makes a 'good eater' plus how to cope with food refusal, mealtime tantrums and fussy eating.

Mealtime behaviour problems are very common

Many parents have persistent worries about their baby's feeding pattern or about mealtime behaviour, with around 13% of babies having feeding problems and at least a quarter of five-year-olds being described as faddy. Even straightforward babies can change and go on to worry their parents over eating as they get a bit older.

There are several broad principles that apply to mealtime behaviour just as much as to other behaviour problems:

- It is always better to reward good behaviour and ignore bad behaviour, rather than rise to the bait.
- Children get confused about rules that seem to chop and change. The clearer the rules, the easier a child will learn them.
- Children very quickly learn where the brick walls are in life, i.e. which rules a parent is never flexible over.
- Children do not automatically know the difference between right and wrong – it needs to be taught. A child is not being naughty if they have never been shown that a particular behaviour is unacceptable.
- Children will do almost anything if it gains attention.

Getting attention is a form of reward

Many children enjoy attracting attention, even if this can only be achieved by being naughty or getting into trouble. Whilst adults may wonder why children should want to be told off, from a child's viewpoint any attention might be preferable to being ignored, and most adults are far more attentive towards a disruptive child than to a well-behaved child who quietly gets on with being good. Hence many parents may unwittingly find themselves warmly 'rewarding' bad behaviour more often than good behaviour, because bad behaviour triggers more attention.

In the general scheme of childhood the best way to learn is by trying things out and monitoring the reaction. The more a behaviour generates an interesting reaction from a parent, the more a child will want to:

- double-check the reaction (by doing the same thing again)
- see how much more of a reaction can be generated by exaggerating the behaviour even more
- see if misbehaving in a different way will get the same reaction
- encourage siblings to do the same in order to see if the parental reaction stays the same or varies.

The above thought processes are not conscious or calculated; it is just the way children tend to find out about the world they live in. The way a parent or other onlooker reacts can override the normal sensations that guide a child's choices, so hunger may go unnoticed if a child is trying to grab some attention from a parent, and the fascination of winding up a parent may be more rewarding than a quiet meal with them.

Even though parents may hate shouting, a child may find it intriguing and be prepared to put up with the noise and long faces just to find out what happens next, how long it goes on for and whether other people in the room join in or are affected. If the parent adds further histrionics, such as banging on the table, bursting into tears, slapping or throwing things (and there are many parents who have been driven to worse by demanding children!), then all these reactions will need to be somehow sorted out in the child's mind. This may well involve doing the 'bad' behaviour again to double-check the reaction it received. In this scenario, a child may feel they have become involved in a stage drama rather than trying to eat a meal, so hunger may be completely forgotten.

When it comes to understanding mealtime behaviour, it helps to see how differently children see things compared to an adult's viewpoint (*see* Box 6.1).

Box 6.1 Mealtime behaviour: how children see things differently to adults

Mealtime factors that bother or interest parents

- Timing of a meal, and the need to move on to other things
- Nutrition
- Cost
- Waste
- Hassle and effort over food preparation
- Mealtime noise
- Mess

Mealtime factors that bother or interest children

- Hunger
- Familiarity of the food
- Flavours
- Interest generated from food
- Parental attention
- Ability to wind up parents over a food issue
- Fun
- Copying what others are doing

In particular, young children have little idea about time. Phrases such as 'teatime will be in an hour' or 'hurry up, we have to leave in half an hour' are meaningless to pre-school children, who will only begin to discover the significance of time as they head through the junior years. They are too young to understand about nutrition, vitamins or the need to eat a balanced diet, but can begin to grasp that some foods can help to keep people healthy, others might cause 'tummy ache', whilst others are simply tasty favourites. Equally, cost and waste are irrelevant – it is flavour, familiarity and interest that count.

Babies who feed poorly

Many babies are simply not fussed about eating, particularly if hunger never really builds up due to frequent small milk feeds. They may find new foods both threatening and strange or possibly rather dull. Food refusal can be most worrying for a parent, creating stress and loss of confidence. Some babies pick up on this, which may occasionally lead on to behaviour problems as a result.

Eating is strongly influenced by feelings, even from a very young age, and parental feelings can sometimes become so intertwined that it becomes difficult to distinguish love and concern from anxiety. In particular, some parents feel a sense of rejection if their child won't eat, as if the child is rejecting the parent's love by refusing to accept food. This can lead to emotional meals, where a parent experiences guilt, frustration and despair, which adds more pressure to the situation.

Babies have a higher risk of eating problems in the following situations:

- prematurity, illness or allergies
- temperament – a child with a difficult temperament may show a tendency to feeding problems from early on
- emotional stress or depression in the mother, as anxieties can be transmitted from mother to baby and interfere with appetite
- problems in the relationship between mother and baby, such as separation – perhaps on going back to work – or difficulties in adjusting to a new addition to the family.

Ground rules for successful weaning

Weaning takes several months and is a gradual process by which a baby gets used to eating a variety of foods, flavours and textures and, even more importantly, learns to enjoy family mealtimes. It doesn't matter about how much is eaten during any individual meal because babies will still obtain most of their nourishment from their usual milk, which is given alongside weaning foods.

- Be confident that a child will get all the nourishment they need from milk, even if starting solids is not going very well.
- Allow a baby to set the pace of weaning, rather than the parent. Babies can get frustrated about food arriving in fits and starts, rather than a continuous flow, and this can override a baby's hunger. By persevering, a baby will get used to the new method, working out how solids need to move from the front of the tongue to the back of the mouth in order to be swallowed.
- Keep calm. Good eaters find mealtimes enjoyable. If a baby notices that

mealtimes produce anxious and stressed-looking parents, then this will reduce enjoyment and may lead to the development of anxieties about food.

- If parents are worried about a baby's growth and find it difficult to relax at mealtimes, then asking a relative or friend to help may improve getting weaning established.
- Refusing food is nothing to do with love. Many mothers feel a sense of rejection when food they have lovingly prepared is spat out or simply refused. Put frustrations to one side, freeze some of the wholesome food and try it again another day.
- For a very reluctant baby, encourage playing with food, squashing and smearing it to explore its texture. As babies usually put things from their hands straight into their mouths, it is likely some will be tried in this way. Parents should be seen happily eating the same food to show that it is nice.
- Some babies learn to tolerate being fed from a spoon by starting with their usual milk being offered from the spoon before moving on to offering solids.
- Just because a young baby scoffs solids with ravenous enthusiasm doesn't mean that it is time for three square meals a day. The process should always be taken step by step because there is a lot to learn along the way.

Food throwing

This tends to be the domain of younger toddlers and is a normal part of development. Babies drop things off high chairs because they can, and the experience of having the item returned turns this into a merry game. All parents play it for a while before informing the tot that 'one more time and I won't pick it up!' It is a game to be enjoyed, but part of the learning process is that games do not carry on forever and babies soon learn that grown-ups will tire more quickly than they do.

Food may be the most handy item on the plate when this game starts, and will form a very educational part of the whole game – toys and teddies are usually returned, but that piece of eggy-bread didn't come back. Why not? The only way to find out is to repeat the process and see what happens this time. As parents tend to react more visibly to dropped food because of the mess, this additional reaction may be exciting enough to inspire further food dropping or even throwing to check out the full repertoire of parental reaction.

A child can be gently taught that this won't be tolerated with a simple 'no' and moving food out of reach. Once distracted, the meal can continue or begin again. If parents react in the same measured way to messy meals then young children will soon learn what response to expect and won't need to keep checking it out.

Youngsters who won't eat

Food refusal in children is common and creates worry for parents. But although children need to eat and food refusal can occasionally be a sign of underlying illness, a poor appetite is often of little significance. Use the flow diagram in Figure 6.1 to assess whether a child's eating tendency should raise concerns and to find out how to help. It requires an idea of the child's usual growth trend rather than a one-off measurement, as described in Chapter 3. This information is usually recorded in the child's health record (the red book in the UK), or the family doctor or health visitor may have it in their records.

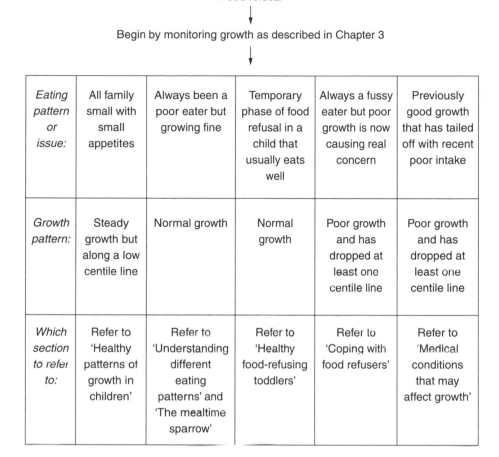

Food refusal

↓

Begin by monitoring growth as described in Chapter 3

↓

Eating pattern or issue:	All family small with small appetites	Always been a poor eater but growing fine	Temporary phase of food refusal in a child that usually eats well	Always a fussy eater but poor growth is now causing real concern	Previously good growth that has tailed off with recent poor intake
Growth pattern:	Steady growth but along a low centile line	Normal growth	Normal growth	Poor growth and has dropped at least one centile line	Poor growth and has dropped at least one centile line
Which section to refer to:	Refer to 'Healthy patterns of growth in children'	Refer to 'Understanding different eating patterns' and 'The mealtime sparrow'	Refer to 'Healthy food-refusing toddlers'	Refer to 'Coping with food refusers'	Refer to 'Medical conditions that may affect growth'

Figure 6.1 Assessing a child who won't eat.

If concerns persist about a child's growth or eating tendencies then further advice should be sought from a doctor or health visitor.

Healthy patterns of growth in children

Some children will be healthily very small and lie along the lowest of the centile lines and others will be healthily large, running along the highest centile line. This is usually governed by genes and may follow family growth patterns, perhaps generating households of beanpoles, petite people or broad-shouldered, stocky children. A child does not need to follow the same line for height and weight; for example, some children will be tall but thin and so follow a high centile line for height but average or below average centile line for weight.

If a family has a distinctive growth tendency then children are likely to follow suit. The centile charts are useful because they show a child's expected growth pattern, which can be reassuring if a child seems a different size and shape to others of the same age. If a child started life on the 3rd centile, then they should continue to roughly follow this line.

In the first few years many children will, on occasion, cross a centile line on their chart. If this raises concern then a general practitioner (GP) or health visitor can monitor growth, but it is often of no significance, reflecting varying growth spurts and occasional illnesses that may upset appetite. It is of more concern if a child veers away from their centile line, especially if the height or weight crosses two or more centile lines. This may reflect poor growth or an underlying problem if growth is too rapid. After a check-up, the family doctor may recommend monitoring the child's growth for a few months to see if the pattern settles down. If concerns persist then they may arrange a further assessment by a paediatrician, particularly if there are other symptoms too.

Understanding different eating patterns in children

The way a child eats is influenced by a series of factors, as outlined in Box 6.2. The two scenarios are extremes and most children will experience a mixture of both good and bad influences, depending on what the day is like and how everyone at home feels. Most children have spells of eating well followed by times when they seem to be off food, which mirrors changes in their rate of growth and sometimes will reflect worries or problems. Growth, natural appetite, worry and illness all affect how hungry a child feels and hence how much is eaten.

Mealtime behaviour, as opposed to how much a child eats, is more related to finding out about how the family functions. Children are always on fact-finding missions that help them understand relationships, and so playing up at mealtimes is a good way to test things out because it is often a time when parents are there to pay attention and to react. Parents should work out whether their child is struggling at meals because appetite is poor or because their child is so busy finding out about interesting aspects of behaviour that hunger has been forgotten.

Box 6.2 Factors that influence the way a child eats

A good eater

- Parents have a laid-back approach at mealtimes.
- Mealtimes and access to snacks are regular and predictable.
- The child has a good natural appetite.
- Parents are confident in the child's ability to make good choices about what and how much is eaten.
- The child finds mealtimes enjoyable.
- Parents set clear boundaries regarding mealtime behaviour.
- The child has an easy temperament and is tolerant of new things and variety.

A poor eater

- Parents feel tense or irritable at mealtimes.
- Mealtimes are unpredictable or food provision is chaotic.
- The child had a poor natural appetite.
- Parents tend to take control over how the child eats, enforcing rules such as clearing the plate.

- The child finds mealtimes stressful.
- Parents chop and change how they react to mealtime behaviour depending on how they feel.
- The child struggles with new foods or too much variety, preferring familiar foods only.

Problems really start when those children with poor appetites decide to test behaviour boundaries because this makes it very difficult for parents to know how to react. If parents are worried about their child's poor growth they may feel far more tolerant of poor behaviour, which then leads on to further testing behaviour because the child has found a first-class way to get attention.

An example that shows the difference between a child with a poor appetite and one who is experimenting with mealtime behaviour is the slow eater. The more slow eaters are nagged, the more slowly they eat. But a child who is experimenting with behaviour will, at their own pace, eat enough for healthy growth even if the process has required 30 minutes of parental chivvying. Parents feel trapped into chivvying because they know that this 'works' in the end and the child eats up. A child with a poor appetite will play with food in the hope that this looks like it is being eaten and because parents reward any effort the child makes with encouraging noises and attention, even though nothing much has been eaten by

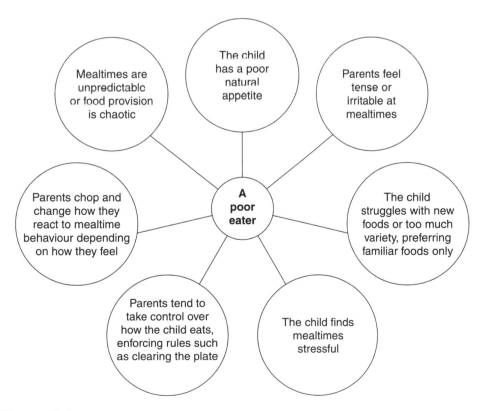

Figure 6.2 A poor eater.

the end of the meal. Again, parents feel trapped into chivvying, despite lack of success, because no other avenue seems obvious.

Alex, at five years of age, was a very slow eater. However, by the end of half an hour or so, if one parent sat with him then he would eat up. His growth was following the expected centile line, although his mother worried about weight loss if he didn't eat up. Both his parents felt trapped into chivvying because they knew it worked in the end and Alex would eventually eat a reasonable amount. Alex loved the attention he received, taking the opportunity to chat about anything that came to mind with his attentive parents.

After Alex's parents were reassured that his growth was nothing to worry about and that he was playing for attention, they ceased the mealtime nagging but gave the same amount of attention in slightly different ways by planning activities to do together immediately after meals. Mealtimes began to speed up because Alex learned that he didn't need to wheedle attention by eating slowly.

Joe, also five years old, hated mealtimes because his mother seemed so stressed about him eating. Mealtimes had become slower over the years. He had learned that she seemed happier if, rather than eating the small amount he wanted quickly, he cut his food into small pieces to nibble with lengthy dawdling and ate only with her encouragement. Joe's mother hated these meals too, but felt trapped into chivvying because of his persistently poor growth on the lowest centile line. She tried hard to hide her disappointment at how little he ate and to show that she was pleased when he ate something, even though it seemed to take forever and never seemed enough to sustain growth.

It dawned on Joe's mum that he was eating to please her. Despite doubts about whether it would work, she began asking Joe to choose what he wanted, which was much less than the amount she usually served, and said she was happy if he ate that. Mealtimes instantly became less strained and because the atmosphere improved, Joe no longer needed to eat so slowly. The vicious circle of worry about mealtimes was also ameliorated, so Joe's appetite began to improve too.

The mealtime sparrow

Some children appear to be poor eaters, but grow beautifully because their overall food intake over each 24 hours is adequate. Whilst each meal seems to be nothing short of a battlefield, calories are on offer throughout the day, so that by grazing and snacking a child can eat what is needed without appearing to take in much food at all. Children may also gain a substantial part of their daily energy from drinks, especially if drinking plenty of milk.

Most mealtime sparrows change how they eat as they get older, with new school routines contributing greatly to this.

Be cautious about the following:

- Is the overall diet well balanced? Whilst a child may be getting enough energy for adequate growth, are there sufficient vitamins, calcium, protein and fresh produce to ensure good health? Consider improving the balance of snacks if they make up a significant portion of each day's intake.
- If mealtime intake is always poor, will settling at school be a problem when the child is less able to graze? Assess how he or she likes to eat, and make small changes that encourage eating in a more formal way, as at mealtimes, to get used to this way of eating. Suggest that snacks are eaten at the table and try to make them form part of a meal, even if little else gets eaten. Move towards limiting food that is eaten away from the table to fruit or safe snacks only (*see* Chapter 13 for more details on safe snacks).
- Avoid mealtime battles whenever possible. Allow children to make choices at mealtimes, such as choosing how much or what type of food is eaten. Stay in control by guiding or limiting what they may choose from, so they get used to choosing, for example, one out of three options, rather than sneering at every one of 15 items in the fridge. Use negotiating tactics to avoid battles over choices by suggesting something be served at the next meal or later in the week if a certain food item is becoming an issue.
- If a child eats like a sparrow, snacks healthily and grows well, stop worrying.

Healthy food-refusing children

This group is a mystery to all but happily the phase is usually short-lived. It usually happens in fits and starts, when every last food is stubbornly rejected, spat out and thrown on the floor. It is really a behavioural problem and may coincide with the onset of tantrums. It may also happen at the end of a growth spurt, when appetite is not so strong. Paying little attention is usually a good thing, whilst continuing to offer food in the usual way. It is quite reasonable to try and make meals interesting, which can be achieved without necessarily pandering to unwanted behaviour. So cut food into shapes, choose colours and textures that are stimulating, and pay no attention to the fact that the child seems to hate foods that once were okay. During this phase it is safe to ignore opinions about liked or disliked foods – right now the child hates everything, but these views will change in time. Continue to offer the usual range of family foods, re-offering new foods over time to generate the familiarity that children need.

The main reassurance during this common phase is the child's milk intake. Milk is highly nutritious and even though it does not contain everything a growing child needs, it will suffice as the main energy source during this passing phase. Be wary of trying to tempt belligerent toddlers with a series of increasingly appealing options, as this is a way of rewarding bad behaviour. Decide what might be a reasonable alternative to the first thing offered, such as a slice of bread or the planned dessert, then, if this is also declined, leave things alone. This approach will not starve a child; it simply guides them through tricky phases by being clear and consistent.

However, a small number of children may develop anxieties about eating, such that the initial short episode of food refusal recurs and, coupled with a naturally poor appetite, begins to affect growth. The following section describes methods for helping children who are not eating enough to allow normal growth.

Coping with food refusers

Fussy eating will often come in phases, but some kids start as they mean to go on and grow into fussy-eating adults! Some insist that all ingredients on the plate are the same colour, or that they won't eat anything they can't peel, or will only eat the white of an egg and not the yolk, or refuse to eat anything with a sauce. Some kids ensure that each mouthful is minute, with each pasta shape eaten one by one, making meals last an age. The list is endless and may change for an individual child over time. Many children simply grow out of it, especially if not too much attention is paid to finicky demands.

Many parents who struggle over food refusal are relieved when their child eats anything, and so are often far more tolerant of snacks and eating between meals. By generating angst and worry at mealtimes, the fusspot discovers the ability to wheedle all sorts of things out of an anxious carer, and may think it is fun to see how many times mum will go in and out of the fridge or kitchen cupboards to offer more and more choice. After an ounce of this, a morsel of that and a sniff of the other, it looks like the child has eaten nothing, but it is enough to take the edge off a poor appetite, with the child feeling safe in the knowledge that they will be allowed to graze later.

Is being fussy a problem?

Obviously this will depend on how pernickety a child is, and whether it affects the overall balance of the diet. Some parents are happy serving the same items in the way their child has come to expect, knowing that the overall diet is adequate even if not perfect. These parents can smooth the transition to school and eating away from home by introducing as much flexibility and variety as possible when in other surroundings.

For those parents who feel their child's fussy eating pattern is an issue, the following questions may shed some light on the root of the problem, and the next section discusses solutions:

- Do tantrums result if the 'wrong' food is served? *This suggests that the child has learned to use food as a method of getting their own way.*
- Does the child simply refuse to eat anything but a very narrow range of foods? *This may indicate a lack confidence and anxiety over trying new things.*
- Despite fussy eating patterns at home, does the child eat with much less fuss for others? *This is suggestive of a child who has learned to wind up parents at mealtimes.*

General hints on dealing with tantrums

Nearly all children go through a phase of throwing tantrums. The terrible twos and tyrannical threes are well named: a tantrum may erupt over the most innocent of stimuli, be immune to the most tempting bribes and happen to any parent in the most awkward situation.

What is going on in the tantrum thrower's mind? Up until the terrible twos, life has ticked by without the child realising that they have a say. When they were hungry, crying resulted in being fed, or when tired, it produced a cuddle or a nappy change. Baby's world has been an ordered pattern of problem–solution, problem–solution.

With growing awareness of the wider world, toddlers begin to learn how to ask for things and to notice reactions and moods, especially of their mother, thus working out that they have some say in the goings on. By testing a few of mum's reactions – for example by crying a little more determinedly – she may act differently, perhaps more quickly or with more concern. This is a huge step forward in life – toddlers learn that they have some control.

Tantrums are a natural progression in finding out the full extent of how much control a child has, and how much effort it takes in order to exercise command over the household. A parent's reaction to a tantrum is therefore important in showing how far this control goes. A parent who panders to tantrums, resorting to anything that will stop the noise, will teach the child that tantrums work. If, instead, a parent pays little attention, perhaps allowing a little flexibility over what the child wants (especially if having a bad day!), then the child will gradually find out that, whilst being an important member of the family, they are not the overall boss of the household.

Of course there are situations where any parent will give in to their child; for example, an awkward public situation, or if the child is putting themselves in some danger, or because the parent has run out of energy that day. But the *usual* reaction is the more important – the one to keep as measured as possible. When tantrums happen in public it is hoped onlookers will politely mind their own business, but if busybodies poke their noses in, a few quips such as 'It's the terrible twos – they won't last forever!' or 'She'll work out who's boss in the end!' will convey who is really in control, even if it doesn't appear that way.

The following suggestions can help the tantrum phase to pass by smoothly:

- Show as little reaction as possible to tantrums. It can be difficult not to react, partly because they are sometimes funny as children fling themselves down and bang their fists, or because they can present a hazard. Whilst taking steps to prevent a child from suffering injury, try not to appear to be joining in the general fight.
- Try to keep reactions the same. As with other behaviours, a child is on a fact-finding mission to work out 'what happens if'. The sooner they work out what the parent's reaction will be to rage and fury, the less it will need to be tried out. If the parent's reaction varies from hooting with laughter to a hearty smack then the child will need to throw many more wobblies to get things straight in their mind.
- Try to say as little as possible during tantrums. Every word spoken during a tantrum is a wasted word. Children are not open to reason mid-outburst so lengthy negotiating is pointless. In fact it may actually reward a child for the behaviour, because talking is a form of attention. Reserve discussions for when things have settled.
- Show some disapproval of the behaviour. This includes hiding a parent's smiles. Little ones can be tremendously funny, and producing a laugh is a great reward for a child, but this will almost certainly mean the behaviour will be repeated. Looking sad and disappointed doesn't require speech. Taking a child to one side or out of the room is a way of showing disapproval by their being excluded.

- Be prepared to sit quietly for longer than the child is prepared to howl.
- Talk about the episode later to ensure the child understands they did not win some sort of battle. Explain that whilst everyone gets cross sometimes, we must learn to control our tempers, and leaving the room or sitting quietly until the outburst fades is one way of learning this.

A plan for dealing with tantrums at mealtimes

Because tantrums can generate a sense of panic in a parent, particularly if there are concerns about how well the child is growing, it is important to have a clear plan to hand. Parents may not need to follow all the steps, but they give ideas about consistent reactions. It might help to put a list of ideas on the fridge as a reminder during the next battle.

- Establish a clear pattern of reaction to a table tantrum. This might involve asking other people in the room to be quiet, so that the tantrum-throwing child can be asked more easily to be quiet too. Some children resort to tantrums just to 'get a word in edgeways' if they live in busy, noisy households.
- Forbid tantrums at the table. This can become a new house rule – tantrums will only be tolerated away from the table. Immediately take the child elsewhere, whether just outside the kitchen door, or the 'naughty step', or bathroom floor – anywhere uninteresting but safe. The aim is to break the association of tantrums with mealtimes, but also it forms a mild punishment because of being excluded from the rest of the family. In addition, it means the family are less able to butt in with unhelpful remarks, which otherwise adds to the confusion that tantrums generate. Even if the tantrum continues in full swing elsewhere, taking charge of where it can take place will show that the parent is in control.
- Once quiet, return to the table unchanged. The aim now is not necessarily to get the child to eat, but just to be quiet at the table. If the tantrum restarts then follow the above step again, and be prepared to do so more times than the child is prepared to throw the wobbly. Most children will settle far more quickly if they are being led out of the room for a second time.
- If parents feel they are running out of energy then announce that the meal has ended and that children may leave the table. If there are concerns that a slight child ate nothing then the next 'meal' can easily be brought forward, even if it means starting again half an hour later. Begin with whatever food seems suitable, perhaps serving the same food again. Once the tantrum has subsided, a child may be happy to eat anything that is provided, because the tantrum was an anger reaction rather than a true objection to the food. Another option is to put a small amount of the earlier food alongside something new, so that the plate looks different.
- Create some choice for children as a way out of a food issue – do not back them into corners by insisting on mouthfuls of food. Suggest either/or options, and state that the food will be served again later or another day.
- Have a fall-back option to remain confident that children will not starve. Make it clear that children are always welcome to eat fruit or a piece of bread, with perhaps a savoury topping, at the end of any meal, regardless of what the behaviour was like during the meal.

- Ask other adults at home to take a similar approach when resisting unreasonable demands from a child. Prevent a child from playing one parent off against the other by discussing together what is acceptable and what approaches the family should take. The rules are less important when a child is out with other adults, such as relatives or friends – after all, everyone gets used to having different rules at home than at work or school, and grandparents are allowed to spoil grandchildren with treats that a parent might not allow. But the rules at home need to be consistent for children to learn them easily.
- Negotiate some neutral ground and compromises. For example, a child might be happy to try one portion or mouthful of a healthy food that will make the diet better balanced if it is with a favourite but less healthy food. Gradually increase this neutral ground to include more variety on the plate, even if it goes untouched. If it keeps on appearing and parents make no issue then one day most children will start to eat some of it.

Understanding food refusers and children who will only eat a few things

This can be a frustrating and mystifying thing for a parent to deal with, but it becomes more understandable when realising that these children are using food as a method of communication. Everyone does it – food as treats, celebration food for visitors, special food when someone has been ill – they are all ways of communicating concern or showing how much people care about and value their friends and family. Food can convey so much more. It is normal for the cook to seek approval when serving a meal, and equally those eating the food will demonstrate whether or not they approve by the things they say, the speed and the way that they eat, or by other signs such as behaviour at the table. But people also convey messages about life in general through food, so mealtime behaviour may mirror general unhappiness.

What is a food refuser trying to say? For young children whose speech is still limited, it will be easier to communicate worry and unhappiness through food than by talking. Some children find the world a frightening place and new foods merely confirm this view. They can cope with fixed routines and the most familiar things, but when these change it makes them feel anxious. Mealtimes, when the familiar favourites appear, are reassuring and comforting. But when new foods appear it can threaten that child's faith in everything else. If familiar foods are not on offer at mealtimes, then does this mean that all the other fundamentals of life are about to change or disappear too? By refusing to eat anything but a narrow spectrum of foods, the child is trying to grasp some control over life. Control the meals and hopefully all the other things in life will stay under control too.

There are many ways to help, as outlined below, but they will take time because they involve boosting a child's general confidence. If children have been through family disruption, or if a child has been affected by being separated from a parent, it may take longer for the dust to settle and for those children to begin to find enjoyment in food.

Occasionally, children begin to refuse food after suffering either illness or trauma that was linked to eating. This may have followed an episode of force feeding (possibly at the hands of a carer who didn't know the child very well), being made to eat when feeling ill so that food seems to have caused the illness, being punished by using food, or perhaps following a bout of food poisoning.

Methods to help children overcome food refusal

Parents who have struggled to cope with their child's very limited eating pattern may have tried endless tactics to encourage eating. Frequently the result is that mealtimes become a battleground with child, parent or both getting upset. For some families this becomes so distressing that meals are dreaded and begin badly even before food is on the table, resulting in a vicious cycle of mealtime anxiety that further hinders healthy eating patterns.

The following ideas can help to break that vicious cycle and encourage calmer and happier meals:

- Food refusers need lots of reassurance that parents approve of the things that the child *does* feel able to eat. In a way, this core food represents the solid ground in that child's life and it is crucial that these basics – as the child sees them – will be there. This means serving favourite foods as the child wishes. Talk about other issues that may be a problem – perhaps a parent has left, or a grandparent has died. Begin to explain that problems such as these are not the child's fault and that the parent's love will always be there, it doesn't depend on how much the child eats and won't vanish even if both parent and child sometimes get upset over things.
- Whilst giving reassurance that preferred foods will be there, talk about adding small amounts of other foods to the plate too, because these are needed for good health. If this is an ordeal, give reassurance that initially these only need to be tolerated on the plate. Work towards actually eating them at a later date.
- When mealtimes begin badly with reluctance to sit at the table, and this pattern is hard to break, try serving favourite meals in different settings – on a tray, in lunchboxes, on a picnic rug, anything that helps to break the association with stress at the table. At the same time, try to do other enjoyable things at the table, such as cutting and sticking, playing with toys, etc., because this will help to associate sitting at the table with enjoyable activities.
- If a child plays up at first sight of a bib then stop using one.
- Show how much a child is valued by asking what they would like to eat, then copying the choice. Talk about how people like to add a few other ingredients to the meal too, to help with staying healthy and because the flavours are enjoyable. Build a firm platform of confidence that what the child is eating is fine, but that it is good to add a few more items for interest, enjoyment, health and sometimes simply because it is in the fridge and needs eating up.
- Begin to make small changes to familiar favourite foods to help the child move towards tolerating more variety. Chop items into different shapes, cook them in a slightly different way, offer varied sauces and ketchups, and combine favourite foods in unusual ways. For example, if bangers and mash or pasta with grated cheese are both popular meals, then try offering mash with grated cheese or bangers with pasta.
- Establish some simple mealtime routines that the child finds reassuring. These routines may help to provide mealtime stability, taking away the need for the food itself to give the child that sense of order and control. Where possible,

establish them a little before moving on to varying the child's food. Examples include setting the table in a particular way, using placemats or particular cutlery and crockery, saying a mealtime prayer together, making a game of washing hands before the meal, or inviting treasured teddies or toys to join in. However, make sure a complex ritual doesn't evolve or life will hardly be any better!

- If, on occasion, the reliable favourite foods are not available, make sure there is a choice of alternatives. Rather than beginning by saying 'We're out of chips, so you'll have to have rice', which will be a recipe for war, consider giving several options, including missing the meal altogether but having extra milk. Other options might include eating something that wouldn't normally be eaten at that time of day, such as breakfast cereal for tea, or the child could be invited to have a look in the cupboard or fridge to see if something else looks appealing. At least by allowing some choice it will be possible to avoid an argument.
- Take opportunities when children are distracted to introduce new foods. Parties and visits to friends' houses are ideal opportunities for adding a few new flavours and textures to a child's plate.

Tips to avoid becoming wound up at mealtimes

It is not only tantrums that get parents fed up at mealtimes. Whingeing, sulking, refusing to sit still, playing with food, ignoring my questions, fighting with siblings: these are a few examples that work in our house. Of course, perfect behaviour from each child at every meal would be not only unbelievable, but rather dull too, both for parents and the kids. Sparring at home is preparation for the wider world and so is an essential part of childhood. Here are some pointers to help parents keep a bit of sanity:

- Parents should recognise their own behaviour at mealtimes. If they are performing fit for the stage, with flailing arms and a megaphone voice, they are the perfect role model for their budding actor children, who will be delighted to copy. If parents need to stamp and shout to let off steam, do it out of earshot.
- Even in the heat of the battle, parents should behave with dignity. They should only use language that they won't mind children using (because again, they will copy), and try to reserve the loudest shrieks for warning of danger only or they will be short of impact when they need a real 'emergency voice'.
- Parents should avoid taking such a firm stand that someone will need to give in. The obvious response from any self-respecting youngster to 'You must eat this!' is 'I won't eat that now if my life depends on it!' Who will win?
- When a couple have different approaches to an issue, they should sort out boundaries together out of earshot of their children. Watching parents argue gives youngsters ideas on how to create mayhem. Watch out for 'Dad said I could' comments. Young children will get confused if parents contradict each other, but as they get that bit older, it will become ammunition!
- Set time limits on irritating behaviour. Kids have very little appreciation of time and won't notice that they have been carrying on for the best part of an hour. They will continue whilst the attention lasts. Parents can warn that if the

behaviour continues for two more minutes then this will result in a penalty, such as asking the child to leave the room, cancelling an expected treat, losing points on a house point chart (if one is being used) or whatever seems to fit the behaviour. If no progress is made after a further one-minute warning then make sure the suggested threat actually happens or parents will quickly lose credibility. Hence it is always a good idea to choose threats that can easily be carried out. There is always a get-out clause if it was a mistake choosing a particular threat, which allows a child to 'buy back' good behaviour. It works along the lines of 'I know you have missed your chance to do whatever it was, but if you now make up by doing the following reasonable task, then we can do it after all.'

- Suggest an alternative behaviour to the child. If a particular behaviour drives a parent mad, rather than simply asking repeatedly for it to stop, divert attention by modifying the behaviour instead of trying to forbid it. A simple example would be to suggest 'If you want to make that noise, could you go and do it in your bedroom?' It is possible to be quite inventive, without appearing to be unreasonable. Suggest challenges, for example 'I can see that you can't keep your bottom still – how about I time you to see if you can keep your bottom in one place for one minute?' or 'Now we've seen who can make the most noise, let's see if anyone can eat their soup without making a single slurping noise.' These diversions usually take the tension out of the situation as well as giving children a new direction to explore.
- If mealtimes are a frequent nightmare, for any number of reasons, then keep them short. Do not ask children to sit down until the food is ready; establish set patterns of expected behaviour before the meal starts to avoid it appearing to begin badly. So, if children should wash their hands before eating, warn them 20 minutes before the meal begins, so it is not a wind-up factor at the start of the meal. If a child always wants to disappear to the bathroom in the middle of each meal then suggest that this happens before the meal starts. For a slow eater, suggest they start the meal a few minutes before everyone else to allow catch-up time, or send other family away from the table for ten minutes to give the slow eater a bit of peace and quiet to finish eating, before inviting everyone back for pudding. If a slow eater is constantly nagged to speed up, it will achieve the opposite, with eating more likely to grind to a halt. Nagging acts as a form of reward for this behaviour because it is attention.
- Let kids eat on their own on occasion. This can be quite a liberating experience both for parent and child. Of course it is inappropriate for very young children to be left alone with food because of the risk of choking, but by the age of four or so, children will find it is fun to eat a meal without a parent's usual running commentary. When little friends come for tea, or simply for a change, serve the meal then disappear. A parent may pop in and out, of course, but the dynamics of the meal will almost certainly alter and children may eat far more straightforwardly when their usual audience is not there to appreciate their antics.

Medical conditions that may affect growth

The commonest reasons for persistent poor eating in young children are usually behavioural rather than due to illness. Difficulties in the home, problems between parent and child, and sometimes lack of knowledge about healthy weaning and suitable foods for young children are fairly common reasons for a child's poor growth. An underlying illness is a less common reason, but should be considered if a child is failing to thrive. A family doctor or health visitor will look into this if parents are concerned.

Medical illnesses that affect growth can be divided into two main groups: conditions that were present and detected at birth, and those that develop during childhood. Childhood conditions are covered in Chapter 15 'An A to Z of conditions that affect eating and weight in younger children'. The following section gives a brief description of problems that appear at birth.

Low birth weight

Some babies struggle to grow adequately whilst in the mother's womb. Before birth, the baby receives all his nutrients via the placenta, so if the placenta isn't working properly then a baby will grow less well.

- Smoking is a significant factor that reduces how well the placenta works and all pregnant women are encouraged not to smoke during pregnancy. Smoking causes narrowing of blood vessels, which is why it can lead to heart attacks and stroke in older people. As the placenta is made up almost entirely of blood vessels, smoking tends to result in it being smaller and working less efficiently. On average, babies born to women who smoke are slightly smaller and are a little more prone to lung problems after birth. If people wish to give up smoking, help is available through the family doctor or through Quitline (*see* Appendix 2 for further information).
- Some drugs have a similar effect, so a woman should check with a pharmacist before taking any medication during pregnancy.
- Pre-eclampsia is another reason why the placenta may struggle to perform well. This is where the mother develops raised blood pressure, fluid retention and protein in the urine during, usually, the later stages of pregnancy. Pregnant women are screened for the condition during routine antenatal checks throughout pregnancy.
- Some infections of the mother can interfere with the baby's growth as can illnesses that affect the mother's own health.
- Multiple pregnancy is another reason why the placenta may struggle to perform well, because it must do twice (or more!) the amount of work. Once twin or triplet babies are born, however, the majority will catch up their growth and reach almost average growth patterns because they are no longer depending on an overstretched placenta for nourishment.

Feeding difficulties at birth

Babies are occasionally born with a deformity of the gut that prevents normal feeding. Whilst in the womb the deformity would not have been apparent because the baby receives all its nourishment through the placenta, and so it may have a normal birth weight. After birth, gut deformities show themselves rapidly with difficulties in swallowing or by causing vomiting, constipation or sometimes breathing problems. Thankfully these types of problems are rare and will be investigated by a paediatrician if suspected.

Genetic (chromosome) abnormalities or heart defects may also be accompanied by feeding difficulties at birth.

There is a variety of illnesses that can cause slower growth in babies. At birth, babies are examined for signs of illness, particularly heart problems, and routine blood tests are offered during their first weeks to exclude conditions such as thyroid disease. With modern ultrasound scanning during pregnancy, some heart defects will be discovered before a baby is even born. A midwife or health visitor can provide further information or leaflets about these tests.

Failure to thrive

As childhood progresses, poor growth may be the first sign of some illnesses, and is called failure to thrive. Whenever there are worries about a child's growth then this should be discussed with the family doctor or health visitor. The doctor is likely to want to monitor growth, usually using the growth charts in the child's health record (the 'red book' in the UK). Where possible, arrange for height and weight to be measured and noted in the child's chart before seeing the doctor.

Chapter 15 covers the common illnesses and conditions that affect weight, growth and ability to exercise in children. Parents who are concerned about their child's growth may find some reassurance by looking at the child overall: a child who is happy, full of energy and growing, even if rather slowly, is unlikely to have a significant problem. A child who is always tired or miserable and showing signs of illness should have a check-up, whether the growth pattern is adequate or not.

Problems of nutrition in the developing world

In some parts of the world there is simply insufficient food to go round due to war or natural disasters such as drought; or there may be poverty so that essential food cannot be purchased or a lack of clean water resulting in chronic diarrhoea and absorption problems. With news broadcasts bringing reports on areas affected by famine, natural disasters or war, pictures of severely malnourished children are not unusual. Severe malnutrition is unusual in the west, but may happen in a child suffering from a severe chronic illness or in a family affected by severe poverty.

A starving child who cannot obtain enough to eat will be at risk of *marasmus*, where all their fat stores have been used up so that muscle has to be used as fuel to keep the body working. The child is extremely thin and gaunt with spindly arms and legs.

Kwashiorkor is a condition where the diet is extremely short of protein, although the child may be fed just enough calories. This causes a bloated tummy and very thin, weak muscles because there is not enough protein for the child to grow properly.

Both types of malnutrition increase the risk of infection.

Summary points

- Attention from parents is one of the most highly coveted rewards for children. It is therefore important to notice and acknowledge good behaviour, rather than encourage bad behaviour by overreaction and attention.
- A child's growth is best monitored over time with several growth measurements rather than a one-off measurement. Growth trends can highlight a problem or give reassurance that the growth pattern fits in with the child's expected growth or family growth trends.
- A tiny appetite is not a problem if the diet remains well balanced and if growth is adequate. Whether a child is a 'good eater' depends on all sorts of things besides natural appetite, in particular a parent's approach to meals.
- Fussy eating may signal that a child has learned to get their own way by using food or it may be a sign of inner worry or anxiety which is being expressed by food refusal.
- Tantrums are a normal part of toddler development, but the phase can be shortened by a calm, consistent and measured reaction from parents.
- Children who will only eat a very narrow spectrum of foods need to gradually build their confidence in general before mealtimes can become more enjoyable.
- Whilst many eating problems are short term and are related to testing behavioural boundaries, there are some medical reasons for poor appetite and failure to thrive.

Chapter 7

Focus on fitness for pre-school children

Changes in our society have made it harder for pre-school children to get as much exercise as in years gone by. Children need to be taught skills to help them take part in sports as they get older and can be motivated to become more active by a combination of parental example and boosting their self-confidence.

Helping young children develop skills to keep fit and healthy

Some of the principles that apply to food choices can also be used to motivate a child to keep fit and active too. Children do not like being forced to do things, but like to do things that are considered fun by other people. They also enjoy doing things that make them feel special, so getting rewards and encouragement will help.

Equally, children will tolerate things that are routine, even if they are dull, so establishing some healthy active norms can help a child keep fit without even realising it. Parental involvement can encourage a child to persist with many activities, but they will soon start to question things if a parent won't consider doing them. Children are not born with the ability to kick a ball, skip or swim, and will benefit from support in both access to equipment and guidance in learning new skills. This increases the chances of their continuing with these activities as they get older.

How much exercise should a child have?

Younger children are better suited to short bursts of exercise throughout the day, rather than one long and tiring session. Some kids will charge about from morning until night with little let-up, but most will prefer intermittent activity, with varied things to try. Overall, a child should aim to take part in moderately energetic activities adding up to one hour, spread over each day. 'Moderately energetic' means enough to be getting slightly short of puff, or feeling as though the heart is beating faster than normal. If a child has not been used to exercising, build up from half an hour in total each day to an hour's activity as fitness improves.

An hour's activity spread over the day might be made up of the following:

- ten minutes' walk to playgroup or nursery, or accompanying older children to school
- ten minutes' playtime on the swings after going shopping

- a game of chase or tag in the living room for five minutes
- an hour's outdoor play, with running and playing on a truck or bicycle counting as 20 minutes of active play
- five minutes' tickling and playing rolling off the sofa
- ten minutes' dancing in front of the television or running about before bedtime.

An alternative way to assess whether a child is active enough is to look at how much non-active play they get. For example, if a child spends most of the day either watching the television, cutting and sticking or doing jigsaws, and feels reluctant to play outside, preferring to go everywhere in the pushchair, there is a good chance that they will not get enough exercise to keep muscles and bones strong and healthy, or get used to keeping active as they get older. However, they might be happy to add in short bursts of activity in between favoured games – these could be gradually increased as strength and interest built up.

Time for older toddlers to walk

In recent decades there has been a change in how parents and carers supervise young children. Years ago, all members of close-knit communities would keep an eye on young children playing in the street and there were far fewer concerns about the risk of traffic accidents or child abduction. Nowadays it is no longer acceptable to leave young children unwatched, which has led to much closer monitoring of where children are and who they are with. In addition, 'shopping' has become more of a leisure pursuit in itself, resulting in children accompanying parents to shopping malls and around supermarkets. Walking in busy and crowded areas raises further concerns about losing children, with the end result that some children spend more time safely strapped in pushchairs than running around. Because the pushchair provides a comfy seat and may also include tasty snacks to keep the child quiet, it is unsurprising that some children are then reluctant to get on their own two feet and walk.

Box 7.1 gives ideas for encouraging older toddlers to walk more.

Box 7.1 Ideas for encouraging older toddlers to walk more

- Avoid trying to pressurise a child to walk, as this will generate 'wind-up' ideas. Try the 'walk a bit, push a bit' approach instead, allowing the child to decide when to swap over. Suggest swapping over at the next lamppost or postbox to encourage reluctant legs to go a little further.
- Invite children to get out of the pushchair to look at interesting things – flowers, insects, shop windows, etc. – in order to discover how much more fun it is to walk and discover the world.
- In safe flat areas and when walking slowly, consider not strapping the child into the pushchair so they can get out easily. However, make sure the child is strapped in properly if walking near busy roads or when walking more quickly to avoid the child being catapulted out if the wheels get caught. Younger babies and toddlers should always be properly strapped in.
- Take a dolly or teddy to strap in instead and encourage the toddler to push the pushchair.

- Leave the pushchair behind – but not if that means having to carry the child instead! Try this on short trips to begin with in case it proves unpopular.
- Pile the pushchair with shopping, etc. so it won't be as comfortable by the end of the trip.
- Plan for the extra time it will take for a child to walk rather than be pushed – do not try this when pressed for time.
- Take a toy pram or pushchair or other push-along toy as this turns walking into a game that many children love.

Taking charge of television viewing

There are good studies to show that simply reducing the amount of time spent in front of the television or playing computer games will increase a child's general activity and possibly reduce the amount of snack foods that are eaten. When watching TV, people tend to sit still and children in particular can become very engrossed in the images in front of them. Other types of play, even doing a jigsaw on the floor, mean a child will move about, reaching, getting up and changing activity far more frequently.

In addition, television provides an engrossing and constantly varying form of entertainment, so that young children will be less inspired to think up their own games and may become reluctant to use the toys in the toy box or go into the garden to play.

Pre-schoolers can be taught to entertain themselves, to think of their own imaginative games using all manner of ordinary household items as well as toys, so that they are less inclined to watch television at the first hint of boredom.

The following tips help to avoid nurturing a pre-school telly addict:

- Create a sense of choice at the same time as limiting the amount of television a child watches. This can be done by suggesting the child chooses between two favourite shows or videos, perhaps reserving the other one for the following day, but not both in the same day.
- Remember that a child has no internal clock where television is concerned. It may be two minutes or two hours later: a pre-school child will be unaware of how much time has been spent watching. Tell children when their TV time is finished, and help them engage in another activity in order to avoid tears.
- Do not worry about using a spell in front of the television as a 'get out of my hair' solution, because children love attention most of all and dislike being fobbed off with situations where they get no attention. Hence this should make watching television less appealing as it will be linked to being fobbed off. The opposite equally applies, in that using television time as a reward will make it appear more appealing, so try not to use this as a bribe.
- Keep a check on the number of hours a child watches each day and try to keep this to less than three hours daily and far less still for children under two. A large study in America showed that hours watching television, particularly at an early age, is linked with attention problems. This study recommended that children under two should watch no television at all, and that older children should keep viewing to less than two hours daily.

- Be aware that television will affect the types of food that a child wants to eat. Another American study showed that for each additional hour a child watches per day, he or she is likely to eat *less* fruit and vegetables, due most likely to these being replaced by foods highly advertised on television. Advertising is a very effective way to make people buy goods, but it is rare to see adverts for simple healthy items such as fruit and vegetables. It is known that the more advertising a product has, the less healthy it is likely to be. Take every opportunity to discuss advertising that is directed at children. The sooner children learn scepticism and to question glossy advertising claims, the better!
- Do not be tempted to put a television in a young child's bedroom. If a special occasion arises, such as a prolonged illness where a child is confined to bed, explain that watching in bed is a temporary thing until up and about again.
- Create house rules so that there is no need to enter into lengthy discussions about TV viewing. Examples might include not watching telly when it's a sunny afternoon or switching off the television at the end of chosen programmes rather than hanging on to see what is on next.
- Avoid settling into predictable routines for watching TV. Because children like routines as a rule, encouraging a pattern of watching certain programmes without fail may result in distress if the routine is broken.
- Watch television with children on occasion, partly to get an idea about the quality of what they are watching, but also to teach them to register if the programme is boring. Unless a child is encouraged to move on to a different activity, they may well sit through dull nonsense without question.

Motivating children to be active

Pre-school children tend to be active by nature, tumbling and trotting as they explore even the simplest things. As they get a bit older, some children begin to slow up and have spells where they consciously avoid anything that seems like effort. Just mention the word 'walk' to a nine-year-old and you might receive a cold stare and belligerent refusal. In order to maximise the chances of an active junior, do some groundwork during the pre-school years.

As with making certain foods acceptable, activities need to appear to be a good choice rather than a lot of unnecessary effort:

- Let children choose from several active options with some 'either/or' suggestions, for example either a trip to the swimming baths, or a game of football in the garden, or going by scooter to a neighbour's to play.
- Activities need to be feasible, which means that a child needs to be capable of taking part. If equipment is provided then it will be necessary to teach the child how to use it before expecting enthusiasm to build up. Be aware of the usual ages that children learn particular skills in order to avoid unrealistic expectations of what a child can join in with. Children start kicking balls from about 18 months of age, but will not be sure-footed enough to kick properly until over the age of three. Throwing is tricky, starting from around two years, but catching is far trickier still, foxing a fair few adults! A child will be able to climb a slide from around two and a half years with supervision, but will need pushing in a swing until at least five years old. Water play will always need

supervision, but there are some super water-spray toys available that are ideal for younger tots, without the safety issues that pools of water raise.

- Activities need to be valued. A child will quickly sense if he is being fobbed off with something boring or unpleasant, or something that a parent thinks is a waste of time. An activity will be more appealing if parents or other grown-ups show that they enjoy it or think it is fun or cool.

- Parents should avoid insisting on games and outdoor play in order to grab a few minutes' peace. Parental attention is highly prized by young children and any ruse that reduces attention will appear second best. Shooing kids into the back garden to give a parent a rest will generate resentment and may make them more reluctant to play outside. Try to get kids absorbed in a game by joining in first, before moving on to get tea ready or doing other household chores.

- Parents do not always need to join in but can show an interest in games, perhaps by offering to keep scores, doing some judicious umpiring and commentating, or by getting the camera out.

- Look at other children of the same age to check if a child is keeping up with skills for games. If a child is reluctant to join in it may be because of a lack of confidence or because certain games appear difficult. Practising ball skills at home is extremely helpful for both the daily activity quota and learning new games, but also for building up confidence to join in.

Boosting a child's self-confidence

Self-confidence is a crucial aspect of a happy life, its significance beginning to count as soon as children become aware that they are part of the wider world. Young children have fears and anxieties just as adults do. It is normal for pre-schoolers to worry about animals and monsters, the dark, going to the toilet and trying new things. They compensate by seeing themselves as big, smart, brave and strong. They do not worry about having to be like everyone else, wearing designer labels or being the winner.

A big aspect of developing confidence is to become a proper member of the household. This means copying what the rest of the family are doing, joining family meals, being encouraged to contribute to family chats (even if that means acknowledging baby babble) or being given a turn at games. They all help a child to work out how important they are in the household and what the family pecking order is.

Particularly if there are older siblings, a pre-school child will be most pleased with being allowed to join in and take turns like everyone else. Complex rules are unnecessary and older children need to be reminded that it doesn't matter if little ones do not play properly, that their score doesn't need to count and that the older children can play to different rules without the little ones even noticing.

For games like football, a pre-schooler will rapidly grasp the idea of practising alone or with a grown-up in order to become good enough to join in with older brothers and sisters. However, if children are always told they are too young or not good enough, this will have a big effect on self-confidence and their enjoyment of the game in general. It is very important for children to feel included some of the time, whatever their skills.

A child who has low self-confidence may be reluctant to take part, tearful and clingy when new activities are introduced or may resort to tantrums, as this behaviour will usually mean the new activity is abandoned. Keep new things as low-key as possible, trying very short spells on lots of occasions rather than a long session. Familiarity will often conquer fear of the unknown, even if the child is still nervous. Build up a child's abilities by doing as many general ball and running games as possible. Get grandparents and other relatives involved where possible. Praise children for trying, perhaps taking photographs as a way of showing a child how proud parents feel.

Little children should start with little games

Particularly in a family with older children, little ones are often left out because they are too young, and then just as they grow up enough to join in, their older siblings grow up and won't play anymore, or, even worse, leave home!

Allow small children to hold the cricket bat, miss a few balls and then realise for themselves that the game is too tricky as yet. At least they will be glad to have been given the chance, will understand why they are not yet on the team, and will get an idea of 'taking turns'. As little children usually have a much shorter attention span too, hopefully older children will understand that this process only takes a moment or two at the start of their games. Often a pre-schooler will be content with having their own plastic version of the kit required for family sports in order to feel part of the family team.

Change and simplify rules as much as needed in order to get pre-schoolers to enjoy games; do not worry about teaching them the correct way to do things – they will pick this up as they get older if they remain keen, but if put off at a young age by complex techniques and rules then they won't even pick up the basics. Playing is how children learn, so guide the process so they can learn more quickly. The aim is not simply to learn how to play a particular game, but to develop strength, balance, co-ordination, patience and a sense of achievement.

Clubs, coaching and home tuition

Now that so many parents have to go out to work, many families struggle to find time for family activities. Most towns have many facilities for children to get involved in a wide variety of activities and this can help busy households. Parents who stay home full time may also benefit from joining local groups or clubs, as this will give access to different toys and sports equipment, plus a chance for little ones to play with other children of the same age. It may be a great way to get to know other mums in the area, or a place to check out worries over a child's general progress by asking other mums who are going through the same stage. Most groups for toddlers are happy for parents to stay for sessions, allowing a child to build confidence whilst parents are in the background.

Good places to find information about local clubs, groups and organisations include the library, local newspapers, the local swimming baths, and notice boards in sports halls or community centres. A detailed listing will be available through the leisure and recreation department at the local council. Health centres and some local church groups may have information about clubs for toddlers and mother-and-baby groups. For families that use a childminder, he or she may be able to take a child to a group on the parent's behalf.

Taking a child swimming from an early age is great for both fun and safety. The sooner little ones develop confidence in the water, the better. Organised swimming lessons may be useful if parents are not able to take children regularly or if they are not confident about teaching children themselves. Many swimming clubs will teach children from as young as three or four years old, but the age that a child starts will depend on their confidence and enthusiasm as well as whether parents have time to take the child along to sessions.

See Appendix 2 for useful addresses of national organisations involved in children's activities.

Parental example – the best there is

Having active parents is a great boost for young children. In studies looking at family activity patterns, it has been shown that having parents who exercise regularly increases the chance that children will follow suit by up to six times.

If parents are considering a fitness drive, doing sports that all the family can join in with, such as swimming and cycling, will be far more inspiring to a small child than if parents disappear off to a gym.

Spending more time out of doors is strongly related to being active, and children will be happier to play outside if parents are involved in some way. Parents can encourage their children to be active by providing equipment, plus ideas and opportunities to exercise, as well as being active themselves and setting an example.

A common barrier nowadays is worry about outdoor safety. Not everyone has an enclosed garden that is safe for young children to play alone in, so this can make it awkward to encourage outdoor play. Cold and wet weather is another common reason for staying indoors, in which case active indoor games can use up a child's energy.

There are options for encouraging active play whatever the circumstances or weather (*see* Box 7.2).

Box 7.2 Options for encouraging active play

Outdoor activity ideas for pre-schoolers

- Sandpit play
- Learning to hit a swing-ball
- Climbing-frame play
- Tricycles, trucks and scooters
- Junior roller-skates
- Skipping
- Building dens – in the garden or on forest walks
- Pond dipping with a net or jar
- Leaf sweeping
- Tending a mini garden or grow bag
- Football, golf and cricket
- Nature hunts – suggest ideas for what to look for, e.g. five different shaped leaves, one insect and three red or yellow things
- Wendy house play – in a real one, or make one with a sheet thrown over the washing line
- Hopscotch

- Wheelbarrow races (hold the child's legs while they try to walk using hands)
- 'Egg' and spoon practice
- 'Tightrope' walking, with the washing line resting on the ground or draw a chalk line on hard surfaces – great for improving balance
- Create a mini assault course with the wash basket, cool box, etc. for the kids to scramble over

Indoor or wet weather activity ideas for pre-schoolers

- Indoor dens – made with anything that won't break!
- Gymnastics or judo on the sofa cushions spread on the floor
- Sliding down the stairs in a sleeping bag (not from the top!)
- Taking teddies on outings to different rooms
- Ball, pool, play centres and indoor climbing areas
- Going to the swimming baths
- Exploring the local garden centre
- 'Large' art projects, using the back of old wallpaper on the floor – this is surprisingly energetic as it involves a lot of getting up and down
- Large cardboard boxes – fantastic fun
- Hide and seek
- Play-mat games
- Strengthen the child's bed so it can withstand being a trampoline
- Rolling bouncy balls down the stairs or a slope – children will run after the ball each time
- Flying paper aeroplanes – again children will want to retrieve the plane
- Dancing
- Dressing up
- Moving around the room without touching the floor

Summary points

- Set pre-school children a good example by getting as much exercise as you can.
- Give children practical help in being active by providing play equipment, opportunities to join clubs or groups, and by helping children to develop the skills needed for games by practising together at home.
- Children will object to being pushed out in the garden just to give parents some peace and quiet.
- Do not make bad weather an excuse to be idle – suggest active indoor games as an alternative to watching television.
- Let pre-schoolers join in with family games to help them learn about taking turns and to boost their general confidence in taking part.

Section 3

Junior children from five to 12

From school age, children begin to understand that health, diet and activity are linked together, making healthy choices more relevant and interesting. Parenting style has a big impact on children; in particular, for children prone to being overweight, there are many positive avenues to improving their health and fitness.

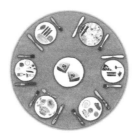

Chapter 8

The healthy body jigsaw

The healthy body jigsaw is a way of putting diet and exercise into the overall picture of what makes people healthy. The more children feel that health is relevant and something they have some control over, the greater the chance they will make healthier choices when parents are not around for advice.

Juniors need information

Between the ages of six and eight years, children gradually change from seeing parents as the ultimate reference point and believing everything a parent tells them to taking on board the views and influences of other people. By age eight, children become increasingly sensitive to their friends' views and what clothes they wear and will pester parents for 'must have' belongings. Eating in fast food outlets is now for status, rather than because the food tastes good.

Even though parents may see far less of their junior-aged children, as they head straight from school to clubs and friends' houses, parents can retain significant influence, particularly if they tune in to how this age group takes information on board. Schooling introduces new concepts to juniors, ideas of self-motivation and finding out things for themselves, and these approaches work just as well at home – better in fact than the overbearing 'because I say so' approach that may have worked quite well for younger children. Lengthy negotiating with a stroppy three-year-old is a fruitless endeavour, whereas negotiating with an informed eight-year-old is more likely to yield results.

Like adults, children from around age eight prefer to do things for a reason rather than because they've been told what to do. It is easier to make good choices if people have learned techniques for making up their minds: understanding reasons behind why a choice might be good or bad is such a technique. Teach children that the easiest route is not always best in the long run. For example, choosing only the tastiest foods may make the overall diet short on essentials and jumping in the car will mean missing an opportunity for keeping fit.

The healthy body jigsaw teaches why and how lifestyle is important, thus boosting commitment and enjoyment from doing the right thing.

Juniors also need information that makes sense rather than mixed messages

Children are bombarded with information – through home, school, advertising and television. What is more, much of this information is complex, too detailed for the age of the child and often simply inconsistent, irrelevant and confusing. Most people suffer from information overload and children can get far more confused than adults. Health messages need to be translated into suitable language for junior-aged children.

A particular problem is giving mixed messages – ones that are true some of the time but not at others. Unless children start to understand why a message can vary in meaning, they will simply learn to disregard messages that appear not to make sense. An example of this is describing a food as 'bad'. 'It's bad for you' is a common expression used about the tasty treats in life, but this gives a mixed message because these are often the most desirable foods or things people consider special. Younger children may initially be worried when seeing their family eating food described as unhealthy, but on discovering that nothing sinister happens – indeed the food is actually enjoyed – they will disregard the 'unhealthy' label and believe what they see instead.

If mixed messages do not end up being completely ignored, then instead they result in guilt. Describing a food as unhealthy by saying it is high in fat or too sugary won't stop people wanting to eat it, particularly if it looks interesting and tastes good. The more exciting and tempting the food appears, the more people agonise over the 'should I–shouldn't I?' question, so that by the time they give in and eat it they feel guilt rather than enjoyment.

An alternative approach is to describe such foods as 'rich' and to teach children that, whilst these foods taste delicious, they are best eaten less frequently than basic foods because they do not fit in well with a balanced diet. Clarifying what is bad exactly about the food, and putting this in context with its good aspects, will help a child understand why we limit some things, so that advice about when it is suitable makes sense. This way, when the occasion is right, rich foods can be eaten guilt-free and with full enjoyment. If rich foods are eaten too frequently then what will be left for people to celebrate with? The Food Frequency Framework in Chapter 13 looks at this in more detail.

There are plenty of mixed messages about smoking and alcohol too

In order to make messages clear to younger children people often oversimplify them – trying to make the world black and white – whereas, for risk-taking behaviours it is more helpful to appreciate the varying shades of grey. For example, whilst 'Do not talk to strangers!' appears clear and suitable for youngsters to take on board, it is less clear when children are asked to answer the front door or buy something from a shop – people talk to strangers all the time in real life. The real meaning of the message is to avoid talking to the wrong kind of stranger – the dodgy sort – but this is rather complex to explain to a seven-year-old, whereas the black and white concept is easier, even if it doesn't always apply.

It is similarly confusing for this age group to see friends and family smoking, which is generally perceived to be dangerous from an early age. Until the age of about 11 or 12, most juniors will strongly object to their parents' smoking habits, applying as much pressure as possible to encourage the parent to stop. A few years later, however, many of those children will have tried cigarettes themselves, often as a result of peer pressure, and then find that the dangers of smoking somehow become more distant and irrelevant to them as an individual.

It is a similar scenario with alcohol. Discovering that parents might drink to excess on occasion may fill a younger child with dread that the parent is an alcoholic, but growing that bit older changes this view, with most adolescents experimenting with alcohol to a degree.

Even though a child may learn a clear health message in school, such as smoking causes cancer and heart disease, this doesn't fit well with the real world where children see many normal, happy and healthy-looking people wandering around smoking. It also raises the stakes of the behaviour – if it is so dangerous then why are people doing it and how come they are getting away with it? It must be worth it somehow.

If people keep quiet about the perceived joys of smoking then eventually many children feel the need to find these out for themselves by experimenting, because it seems plain that there must be some benefit, and, what is more, the risks seem invisible. A child will form a better understanding if the good points as well as the bad are discussed, in order to weigh things up without necessarily having to find out half the story from personal experience.

A few food issues that confuse children (and adults!)

Table 8.1 lists some of the food issues that may cause confusion or send out mixed messages.

Table 8.1 Some food issues that contain confusing or mixed messages

Food issue	Confusing or mixed message
References to cholesterol	This complex term will be meaningless to a child unless they study it as part of a GCSE course or similar. Do not bother mentioning it to children under 12.
Is fat good or bad for people?	A healthy diet should contain up to 30% fat so there is only a problem when there is too much fat in the diet. Vegetable oils are healthier than fat from animals.
'Health-giving' foods	Eating 'good' foods (such as special yoghurts) will not undo the damage that too many rich foods might cause. The only magic ingredients that will restore the balance of a diet short of fruit and vegetables are fruit and vegetables.
Are vegetables really healthy?	A child may be forgiven for finding this hard to understand if, until now, vegetables have merely been used as a threat at mealtimes! Facts that may be obvious to an adult may be far less clear to a child.
Will added vitamins make a food healthy?	Added vitamins may slightly improve the nutritional value of a food, but won't remove the excess fat, salt or sugar that it contains. Just adding a few vitamin drops to a rich food will not make it suitable for frequent consumption.

The healthy body jigsaw

Figure 8.1 shows how to help children understand health issues.

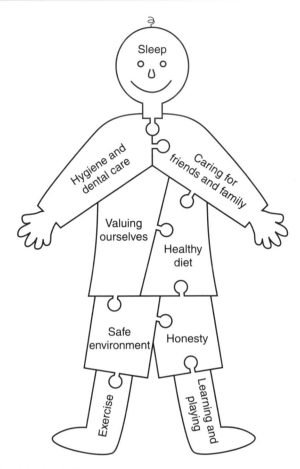

Figure 8.1 The healthy body jigsaw.

When starting school, children get used to dealing with separate subjects that link together. If children are reluctant to change to healthier lifestyles, they can become more interested by discovering the wide variety of things that keep people well: improving any area can make a difference to health in the long run.

To begin with, people need a balanced diet with plenty of fruit and vegetables, and milk to help bones grow. Exercise helps to strengthen bones, keeps muscles in good shape and keeps the heart healthy. Watching TV is good for enjoyment and quiet relaxation, and working hard at school will give extra brain power. Sleep is needed for brains to recharge, rather like a rechargeable battery.

In addition, it is important to keep the environment healthy too – which means tidying up litter, not leaving toys on the stairs where someone could trip over them, and closing gates and doors to stop toddlers running off. And what about emotions? People feel happier when they value their friends, when they are truthful and when they take the trouble to share. In particular, looking after family and listening to them if they are worried increases the chance that they will do the same when it is our turn to be down.

Getting the balance between all these factors right is fundamental because everything can go askew when one piece of the jigsaw is missing. Families may be able to think of more jigsaw pieces that apply to their household.

When all these elements balance each other it leads to good self-esteem, which means having a good view of oneself. This in turn produces self-confidence and inner strength so that it is easier to make good long-term choices. If elements are neglected then it puts the person's overall health at risk, either in the short term or in the long term. The following section looks at each element in turn.

Safe environment

This incorporates both the physical space that we live in and the ideas that guide our lives. For example, imagine the dangers for a child crossing a busy road in the rush hour without any knowledge of traffic safety. For the child to cross safely they will need to know how dangerous it is to run in front of moving vehicles, plus how to find a zebra or pelican crossing, or, if younger, then not to cross the road at all unless with a grown-up. Just as much caution should apply to a child walking through a busy shopping centre with a purse full of money. It will be useful to understand the value of money in order not to be ripped off, simple safety about hiding valuables so they do not get pinched, not talking to strangers unless they are there to help (such as shop assistants or policemen, etc.) and also what purchases are suitable. Many items in shopping precincts are tempting, but that doesn't mean that everyone should buy them all.

Some parents are happy for their children to choose for themselves how much confectionery they eat, but this is unfair on a child who has not been made aware of the dangers of eating too much, in the same way that it would be unfair to leave a child merrily pulling a cat's tail without warning them that the cat may bite and scratch when it has had enough taunting. If children are unaware that frequent sweets and crisps may cause at the very least tooth decay, if not illness, then there will be little motivation to leave them aside.

Living in a safe environment means learning to be aware of all the hazards that surround us, as well as which things are safe, so that children are able to make informed choices as they grow up.

Sleep

No one really understands why people need sleep, but all mammals and most other animals seem to need it. A koala bear spends 18 hours a day fast asleep, whereas the giraffe gets by with a mere 20 minutes. Ducks even sleep with one eye open, resting half of their brain at a time, so that they can keep the other eye out for danger. A rat will only live for a couple of weeks if it is starved of food and the same applies if it is starved of sleep. It is something we cannot do without.

Human adults need around eight hours' sleep each night, but children need more. Teenagers really need about nine hours to function well and juniors need ten (although this varies for individual children). Babies spend most of their time asleep, up to 18 hours or so for a newborn, but this gradually gets less over the first few years as daytime naps are dropped.

Sleep is a time when the brain 'recharges its battery' and a lack of sleep causes all sorts of problems ranging from memory lapses to accidents, moodiness and behavioural problems. Many children become agitated and hyperactive rather than sluggish when they are tired.

Giving children a calming down period of 15 to 30 minutes before they are expected to go to sleep will help them settle. Watching television just before bedtime is a way of stimulating the brain, making it harder to fall asleep. Try quiet reading or a board game instead. Children can be encouraged to help with tidying and to think about the next day as a routine before bedtime, as a way of 'putting the day to bed' and getting ready to sleep.

Honesty

Being honest and trustworthy is not usually linked with being healthy, but both are important for mental health. It feels good to be trusted and it often brings out the best in people. When a person is relied upon they feel valued, and children will often surprise adults by how seriously they take a task if its importance and value has been explained.

Trust in others is essential for the world to work. Imagine trying to do the shopping if the shopkeeper can't be trusted to weigh things correctly or if the packet says six cakes but contains only four. Because people can't know everything themselves, they have to trust others, so if the car mechanic says the car needs a new crank shaft, most people have to take his word and trust he is telling the truth. If the doctor says an operation is required, then people hope and trust that it is the right decision.

How do people know that it is okay to trust all these people? It comes from knowing that we ourselves are trustworthy. Learning the difference between right and wrong is as basic as learning to read and write. When people show respect to and trust in others they usually receive the same in return. Being lied to is painful and being discovered to have told lies creates a feeling of shame. Mental health and happiness are greatly affected by whether people can be trusted and can put their trust in others.

Caring for friends and family

Although the concept of 'survival of the fittest' might make selfish behaviour appear better for survival, humans are in fact team players. People live in communities rather than as isolated individuals, and this means learning the rules that the communities follow. Selfish people who pay little attention to community rules find it difficult to integrate, and so it is important for children to learn customs and traditions so they can fit in. Many aspects of childhood are geared to learning this, such as taking turns, losing graciously, sharing and saying sorry.

Most children find the process hard work to some extent and the more parents allow children to think of themselves as the most important person in the household, the harder it is to learn to care for others. One consequence of parents devoting themselves to their children is that those children will, in return, care for their parents once they have become elderly. Children can be taught that by looking after friends and family, they are ultimately investing in themselves.

Valuing oneself

It is easy to have good intentions, to plan to make new changes and give up bad habits, and to aim high. However, carrying out those good intentions, achieving goals and sticking to new regimes require an essential ingredient, motivation. There needs to be a driving force behind not only *wanting* to do something, but actually *doing* it.

Where does motivation come from? One of the most important things that stimulates motivation is valuing oneself, the sense of knowing that we are worth making an effort over. When people feel bad about themselves it is hard to make the effort to do healthy things. Who, after all, bothers to look after what they think is rubbish? Box 8.1 lists some factors that make a difference to whether someone feels motivated or not; these will vary depending on the task in question.

Box 8.1 Where does motivation come from?

- Self-respect, which makes the individual feel that any effort will be worthwhile.
- Inspiration from others, especially teachers or specialists in a field, such as sports stars.
- Interest and enthusiasm, which will depend on the topic.
- Knowledge of the benefits that can come from working on a topic.
- Spur or stimulus due to fear of failure, or knowledge of the problems that may arise if the topic is neglected. (An example might be the spur to stop smoking after seeing a relative die from a smoking-related illness.)
- Incentives, such as rewards for achievement.
- Inner drive, which usually stems from an individual's personality.
- Following the example set by friends or family, because it feels good to join in.

Motivation will be in short supply unless there are obvious benefits that make something worth a try. Take the example of eating fresh vegetables: to begin with a child will need to know why they are essential – because they contain lots of goodness such as vitamins, minerals and fibre, but no harmful ingredients. They taste wonderful once a person becomes accustomed to their flavour and texture. Top athletes will eat masses of fresh produce in order to boost their sporting abilities. Insufficient vegetables can lead to health problems such as constipation and poor growth. When people enjoy fresh produce they will find more enjoyment from interesting menus in restaurants or when visiting other people's houses. Even if vegetables taste unusual or strange to begin with, by trying small amounts on a regular basis, they will soon become familiar and tasty.

What about motivating a child who is overweight?

From as young as seven years of age, children are aware of body image and the effect it has on others. It is a sad fact, and one that is picked up quickly, that overweight children are often teased or bullied, and even some adults may treat them less fairly. Overweight children therefore often have a very negative body image and generally low self-esteem. Because others appear not to value them, they have less value in themselves. This then makes motivation to do healthy things much harder. Obese children may want to be healthy, but the incentive to feel that the effort will be worthwhile is not there.

Improving a child's view of themselves and practical ways to boost motivation are discussed in detail in Chapters 10 and 11. By building up a child's self-esteem and self-respect first, further changes to lifestyle will become more achievable.

Learning and playing

Play is the main route by which children learn, whether it is dressing dolls in preparation for their later role as parents, or taking part in games and sports. Children do not play just for fun, but to build up strength, co-ordination and balance, and to learn skills, communication and the way that their community works – its customs and rules. Although children are able to learn by instinct, they will learn more efficiently if they have guidance along the way.

Children who find enjoyment from learning new things will find the world a fascinating place. This enjoyment will be boosted if parents show enthusiasm for their interests, support their attempts to make and do things, and teach skills so they are picked up more easily than if left to struggle alone. A child's play is as important as an adult's work, and it is a crucial foundation for later abilities as an adult. The more varied the play opportunities a child has, the more skills will be picked up along the way.

Hygiene and food safety

In times gone by, an average man or woman would have been lucky to live beyond their forties. But in the last 150 years, the average life expectancy for a woman has increased to 80 years and for men to 75 years of age. Many factors have helped people live longer, such as safer working conditions, better nutrition and healthcare, but a significant one has been improved hygiene so that people are less prone to serious infections.

Being clean doesn't come naturally to children, so they need to learn basic hygiene house rules, as outlined in Box 8.2. Looking after teeth is discussed separately in Chapter 15.

Box 8.2 Examples of hygiene house rules for children

- Wash hands before touching food.
- Only use clean spoons to serve food that is to be shared, rather than a spoon that has already been licked.
- Do not lick the lids of containers that still contain food.
- Keep feet off tables that will have food served on them.
- Do not eat food that has been dropped on the floor where there are germs and dirt, unless it can be washed.
- Always close the fridge or freezer door or else food inside could go off.
- Check the temperature of each mouthful of hot food to avoid burning the mouth.
- If poorly with a tummy upset, use a separate towel and kitchen utensils from other members of the family.
- Put a hand in front of the mouth before coughing or sneezing.

- Use a handkerchief or tissue for a runny nose, rather than a sleeve.
- Boys should lift the loo seat before peeing.
- All children should flush the loo after a visit and then wash their hands.

Simple measures are very effective at reducing the risk of catching infections, particularly gut infections, and all children should be reminded regularly of usual hygiene rules until they become habit. Introduce further ideas as children get older, such as checking 'use by' dates and which food should be kept fresh in the fridge to avoid it going off and causing tummy upsets.

A healthy diet

The first two chapters discussed how a child could be guided towards enjoying healthy foods and be helped to recognise when full. Many parents may find this hard to put into practice because they have already found that their children enjoy and demand either a very limited range of food or junk food. This section looks at ways to motivate a child to question the things they have liked until now and to broaden tastes so that healthier foods become more acceptable.

This process involves:

- providing information about food
- supporting children by parents picking up on healthy ideas that their child suggests, and by finding practical ways to boost enthusiasm when it wavers
- questioning parents' assumptions about what foods their child likes – children may have healthier tastes than we think.

Providing information about food

This involves teaching children to understand the information that is all around us, as well as finding sources of information that a child may find interesting.

Discuss the basic ingredients of a healthy diet by referring to *The Balance of Good Health*, as described in Chapter 1. Ask children if they can put their favourite foods into the appropriate categories. Try and work out together if the usual diet is well balanced or if there are too many of some foods and not enough of others. Parents do not need a detailed knowledge of nutrition for this because *The Balance of Good Health* is simple to use.

Junior-aged children respond well to challenges and a good one is to ask whether they have had their daily quota of at least five portions of fruit and vegetables today. (Perhaps do this before the last meal of the day has ended in case more are needed.) See Chapter 12 'Nutritional nuts and bolts' for further details on portion sizes and which foods count as fruit and vegetables, because not all produce falls into this category. For example, potatoes are classed as a starchy food rather than as a vegetable.

Nutrition information is now printed on the packaging of many items of food. However, it is usually in small print and may make little sense to people who are unfamiliar with it. When shopping with slightly older children, perhaps in the holidays, try looking at some regular shopping purchases to see what information is provided, to become familiar with the terms used. Some ideas of what to look for are given in Box 8.3.

Box 8.3 Ideas for making use of the nutritional information box on food packaging

- Compare the calorie content of similar-looking products, for example a tomato sauce for pasta, perhaps comparing a brand leader with the supermarket's own brand. Look at the 'calories per 100 grams' for each product because this will show which is lower in calories, regardless of whether the two jars are the same size. Variations are usually due to the amount of oil used in the sauce, even though they may taste very similar. The lower calorie option is usually healthier.
- Find out how much fibre per 100 grams an item contains compared with other similar products. This is useful for comparing breakfast cereals and types of bread. If children are prone to tummy pains due to constipation then moving to a higher-fibre breakfast cereal is a simple solution.
- Is a food unnecessarily sugary? When trying to encourage the family to cut down on sugary foods, taking a look at the carbohydrate content can give an idea of how sugary each is. Carbohydrates are listed as follows:
    Carbohydrate . . .
    Of which sugars . . .
  If the listed sugar makes up more than half of the total carbohydrate amount then it is a very sugary food. Look for similar products that have a lower ratio instead.

Without worrying children unduly, explain that diet can affect how prone people are to illness, particularly as they get older. Junior children have a very limited understanding of different illnesses, but can begin to understand that eating too many fattening or sugary foods or getting insufficient exercise leads to diseases of the heart. Many children in this age group begin by thinking that 'heart disease' or a heart attack is due to being sad, as in a broken heart, and do not realise that the heart is the organ that pumps blood around. Unless this is made clear then a child may struggle to understand why apples and broccoli should stop a person feeling sad after a divorce or bereavement!

Let children discover things for themselves

Many adults will remember a childhood trip to a sweet or cake shop and the sensation of feeling spoiled for choice, but then the disappointment of finding that the final choice was not that great. Perhaps the experience was in a toy shop, when following lengthy agonising, the chosen toy fell apart within hours of its purchase. It is a valuable lesson to learn, along the lines of 'All that glisters is not gold', and it applies to food because outward appearances can be deceptive in terms of both flavour and health. Children learn this far more quickly if allowed to make a few mistakes, rather than being told not to try things without ever having the chance to test the evidence. A child who has made themselves sick by eating too many sweets is likely to remember the lesson.

Parents can support children by picking up on healthy ideas that their child suggests, and by finding practical ways to boost enthusiasm when it wavers

Discussing the balance of a child's diet together will show what they think about food in general:

- Are they bothered or uninterested?
- What about trying new things?
- What about the concept of reducing their intake of less healthy foods and eating more of the healthy ones?

If children are involved in changes to family lifestyle there is a greater chance of their going along with new ideas. If they also have their own suggestions as to how the family might eat more healthily, these changes should be tried even if the change is very small. As children learn more, good ideas will grow and enthusiasm will be far greater if they know they will be listened to.

If a child seems uninterested in eating habits, for the meanwhile focus on other parts of the human body jigsaw instead, such as getting plenty of exercise. Revisit food issues at a later date.

If a child agrees that the current diet is not good enough then explore new foods together. Buy small quantities of new things to reduce the chance of waste and look for several recipe or serving ideas so that the new food has a proper chance, because people often grow to like things once they are familiar.

Following a cosy chat, many kids profess great enthusiasm for new ideas, but several days later have already forgotten that a change was even mentioned. If, for example, both parent and child agreed to limit crisps to alternate days, it would be no surprise if the child began moaning by the second crisp-free day. Talk again about the good reasons for improving everyone's diet and give some flexibility about carrying it out, without giving up on the idea. So, continuing with the same example, suggest getting used to smaller quantities by putting half a packet of crisps in a smaller container and having occasional crisp-free days first before reducing them further. At the same time, focus on the healthy foods that *are* being eaten and encourage every opportunity to 'take five'.

Avoid making a big issue about sticking to new plans or initial enthusiasm may change to hostile refusal if children sense that they are now being backed into a corner. Going on about an issue is usually a good way to give a child 'wind-up' ideas. Instead, try to keep positive health issues part of family conversations so that children gradually pick up new concepts by the 'little and often' approach.

Parents should question their assumptions about foods they think their child likes — children may have healthier tastes than first imagined

Some surprising results came from a large French study, which asked 1000 nine to eleven-year-olds and their mothers about their views on food and eating. The first finding was that children see food as a necessity of life, whereas mothers view food mainly as a pleasure for their child, with necessity and nutrition given lower importance. This should reassure mothers that mealtimes do not have to be opportunities to curry favour from their children — they're just expecting a meal rather than entertainment and any old food will be okay as long as it tastes reasonable.

When planning a varied diet, 'variety' means eating foods from the different food groups throughout the day, rather than eating different flavours every day. The same well-balanced meals can reappear time and time again as long as they have good proportions of fruit and vegetables and starchy foods, plus protein and dairy items. If well-balanced meals become familiar then they will often become favourites and a major hurdle of childhood will be solved.

The second finding of the study was that, contrary to popular belief, children's enjoyment of 'unhealthy' and 'healthy' foods was similar. French fries were the most popular food for 92% of children, closely followed by pasta (89%). Fruit and candy (or sweets) received similar scores of 82% and 81% respectively, which really begs the question of why children eat far more sweets than fruit when both are popular. It may suggest that cost and convenience play more of a part than enjoyment, plus parents may wrongly assume that their child doesn't like fruit and so leave it off the shopping list.

The third finding showed an increasing trend for watching television during mealtimes, with 25% of breakfasts and over 40% of afternoon snacks and evening meals being eaten in front of the TV. This has important consequences for family eating: television distracts viewers from noticing fullness cues, resulting in more food being eaten; there will be exposure to advertising of unhealthy foods and a reduction in family networking, when family values are established.

Parents should review their ideas about which foods their child likes and dislikes and test out new ideas. This study commented that many mothers found it difficult to combine the demands of family life, working, healthy eating and keeping mealtimes pleasurable. It is not an easy balance to get right, but perhaps it is not quite as difficult as we have led ourselves to believe.

Making exercise relevant

For children to be active, games must be likeable as well as do-able. Part of the motivation for exercising comes from knowing why it's a good thing, so this section discusses why exercise is healthy.

There are a great many children who need no encouragement to be active; it is simply a childhood certainty. But as children hit puberty and move on through the teenage years, the tendency to partake in sports often dwindles or vanishes completely. Understanding how exercise helps the body may help children to see that in addition to sports being fun, they are a vital part of being a healthy human. If the fun element fades with the onset of puberty, this knowledge may help a child persevere with some activities.

Exercise builds up strength

Although obvious to adults, a child may not realise that exercise will build bone and muscle strength, as well as keep the heart healthy and reduce the chance of becoming overweight.

Unlike toys, which tend to fall apart if they are overused, bones and muscles love to be used. The more use they have, the stronger they become. When a person is unfit, muscles scream if they are exercised hard, but thankfully these muscles soon get used to new activities if done regularly.

Astronauts in space face a real problem with not being able to run about or even walk. Unless they do lots of gym exercises whilst in space, they find that their leg muscles literally waste away, making their legs spindly and weak, because the muscles are not being used. The way to build up muscle strength and bulk is to keep exercising them.

Exercise keeps our insides clean

Exercise makes muscles stronger, and because the heart is made of muscle, getting fitter will make the heart healthier. Further, forcing blood to flow faster through blood vessels is one way to keep them clean. Blood vessels – the veins and arteries – are rather like long drainpipes which can get clogged up with debris and rubbish, especially if the diet contains too much fat. It is not possible to give them a good scrubbing with a brush so they need cleaning differently. Water forced through a pressure hose would work on a sludgy drainpipe, and vigorous exercise, such as running or dancing, has a similar effect on blood vessels because the increased blood flow helps to clean rubbish off the walls. It must be energetic exercise that leaves the person out of breath and with the heart racing.

At the same time, do not eat too much 'rubbish' either, so that blood vessels are less likely to get clogged up to begin with. Eating too much fat not only makes people fat, but clogs up their insides too.

Exercise stops people from storing too much fat

Even though surveys show that children today eat fewer calories than they did 50 years ago, far more of today's children are overweight. A major reason behind this is the trend to be far less active both in terms of the way children play (think of computer games and television, which were not around then) and because of the lifestyles we lead. Most households now have access to a car, use a variety of household gadgets to reduce manual tasks and have some form of heating so that there is no need to use up as much energy in keeping warm.

If a child enjoys a very rich diet and is reluctant to change it, then being more active ensures that the excess energy eaten is burned up by busy muscles, rather than stored in fat cells, which may lead to a weight problem.

Exercise makes people feel good

Think of the rainy day blues, those listless days when everyone feels bored. We all cheer up when the sun comes out because we can get busy doing something again. Busy children do not complain of being bored.

Some people take this to extremes with endurance sports such as marathon running. They choose to do this for pleasure because they enjoy the activity and how they feel at the end of it, even when exhausted, and because of the sense of achievement. When people exercise hard the body releases a special substance called endorphin. It is a bit like an inbuilt painkiller and gives off a feel-good factor, so that some people love exercising because it makes them feel great.

Summary points

- Children love information that makes sense. Explain why some 'mixed messages' can have two different meanings so that children do not learn to ignore them entirely.
- A safe environment means appreciating the varied hazards around us and understanding that whilst many things are okay in moderation, they can be harmful in excess.
- Honesty and trust have surprising effects on emotional health because of their positive effects on self-esteem. Learning to take turns and say sorry helps children to fit into their community.
- Children need to feel they are worth making an effort over in order to make good choices. This means learning to value and care for themselves as well as their friends and family.
- Hygiene is a basic part of good health and all children should be reminded regularly of hygiene house rules until they become second nature.
- Help children to find out how healthy their existing diet is using nutritional information and *The Balance of Good Health*. Encourage their ideas on making improvements and make health a routine topic of discussion.
- Children do not expect grand feasts on a daily basis; ordinary foods are fine most of the time. Many children enjoy healthy foods just as much as less healthy ones.
- Explain why exercise is beneficial so that children feel any effort they make is worthwhile.

Chapter 9

How does parenting style influence children's behaviour?

There may be a hundred ways to kill a cat, but there must be many thousands of ways to bring up children. Some parents fuss, others do not; in some families both parents spout the same ideas, whereas in others there are varying views from each member of the household. Whether strict or laid back, anxious or confident, consistent or prone to changing the rules, all these factors will have an effect on mealtimes.

This chapter takes a look at four aspects of parenting and how they affect childhood behaviours:

- a parent's level of confidence
- parental awareness of a child's diet, body shape and size
- how food is used to communicate with children
- the mechanisms that are used to teach children about eating.

Confidence in parenting

The confidence that parents have in how they bring up their children comes from a combination of personality, their own upbringing and the reactions they get when trying an approach. Some parents find the child-rearing task to be one long, agonising worry, in which they lurch from anxiety over one issue to indecision over another. Other parents make snap decisions without any appearance of uncertainty and may seem to rule over their children with a rod of iron. The majority of people sit in between these two extremes, worrying over certain issues, such as how to reduce the amount of TV that children watch, but taking a more confident line over others. But what effects do the two extremes have on children?

Indecisive worriers

If, as can sometimes happen, a parent loses all confidence in making decisions, then the child will pick up on this and start to question other things that the parent says. The resulting conflict leads the child to become unco-operative, and with every parental request or comment now being challenged, further doubt fills the parent's mind over how best to handle each situation. As time goes by, with more decisions challenged or ignored, the resulting clashes worsen the parent's confidence, thus making decisions even harder, creating a vicious circle that allows the child to take control.

Sam, at age nine, was a bit of a telly addict. His mum, Alison, was concerned as she had noticed 'spare tyres' around his tummy, and he no longer fitted into clothes suitable for his age. Sam enjoyed his food and Alison wondered whether to try and get Sam to be more active, rather than tackle his liking for junk food.

She talked to Sam about the need to get healthy and said that from now on he should limit his TV time to two and a half hours a day, rather than the four to six hours he was used to.

Sam initially ignored her comments, but when she gently tried to enforce the plan, he accused her of nagging and then went to lengths to destroy the other games she had suggested he might play with instead. The final straw came as Sam screamed at her, 'And don't even try stopping me eating chips!' She now felt certain that she couldn't face a similar battle to try and improve Sam's diet.

Sam's behaviour seemed to get worse, even though she backed off from commenting on how much TV he was watching.

In this situation children often wish for clear advice, to feel they can rely on the parent, but are frustrated by their own doubt in the person they want to trust. This produces a defiant and sometimes aggressive child, but one who is strangely enough very reliant on the parent. The parent is increasingly criticised by the child, at the same time as being expected to make decisions.

Alison discussed her worries with another parent, Penny.

'It looks like you walked onto a battlefield as the weaker army, lost the battle and now he's taking prisoners. What's more, he hasn't suffered at all for the fight,' Penny volunteered. 'The only way I can get new plans past my kids is by going for hefty incentives. Link giving him pocket money with TV time – full money only if he keeps within the limits five days a week, and reduce the amount a bit for each day he's over. He'll start to think it might be worthwhile if he finds himself losing out. It might be bribery, but at least it's a language he'll understand.'

Alison planned out these ideas, gritted her teeth and presented the new positive plan to Sam. She was quite shocked to find that, after keeping quiet initially, he told her exactly what he had earned by the third day of the new regime.

Sam had sensed that his mum meant business, but also that the new plan seemed worth a try because it came with a suitable carrot.

On the one hand, it is good for children to be involved in making choices about their lives, but on the other, seeing a wavering parent may give a child wind-up ideas, or a desire to test the parent to see what reaction he gets from refusing to comply.

It is best for parents to keep uncertainties out of earshot until they have decided which options are suitable for the child to choose from. At this point the child can become involved in having a say because all the proffered choices have some merit, so the exact choice is less crucial and the parent is clearly in ultimate control.

The rod of iron

Forceful parents can end up with equally forceful offspring, but it is more likely that children of such parents might feel timid and hesitant about making their own decisions. This is because children need to practise making choices, but if not given a chance to do so because their views and wishes are overridden on a regular basis, this dismissive approach will knock self-confidence and leave the child feeling worthless and undervalued.

Many parents believe that forbidding or putting limits on their child's access to certain foods will help their child not to want that food. But surveys reveal the opposite; once parents are out of the way, those foods become top choices, which are more likely to be overeaten.

Being dogmatic and inflexible about letting children make up their own minds ultimately leads to them choosing exactly the opposite of what their parents had in mind. Kids need to find out for themselves, and if they do not do so in childhood, then they will make their mistakes later on in life when they do have control and may be more likely to stick to unhealthier lifestyles in an act of defiance.

How aware are parents of a child's diet, body shape and size?

The current 'obesity epidemic' has almost crept upon us unawares. Because there is no clear cut-off between being about right and carrying a little too much weight, it is difficult to know when to take action. It is not like a rash – obvious when it's there and plain when it has gone. But the evidence suggests that parents are not even worrying when things are serious. In a UK survey by the Earlybird Diabetes Project, where 20% of a sample of seven-year-old children were overweight or obese, they found that most parents felt their kids were about right, failing to recognise a weight problem in one-third of girls and half of boys. They also discovered that 40% of parents with obese children and 75% of parents with overweight children were not concerned about their child's weight.

If people are unaware that there is a problem it becomes even harder to find solutions.

Unfortunately, once an overweight problem sets in, it is hard to treat. At least 40% of obese children will remain so as adults; and with obesity becoming commoner and more pronounced in children, this percentage might well worsen.

Rather than upsetting children, making them aware of health issues and developing problems at an early age is of benefit, when improving lifestyle is not seen as such a big deal and when it will be more effective.

Ignoring the facts introduces denial

There are all sorts of ways of ignoring weight problems. Comments such as 'It's puppy fat', 'He's a growing lad' or 'She has big bones' are commonly used to help overweight people feel that there is a perfectly reasonable excuse for their shape or size. Much as it is good to reassure children that they are healthy and that we love them however they look, it is unhelpful to do so to the extent that potentially serious problems are brushed under the carpet. Allowing a chubby junior to progress into an overweight teenager and then on to an obese adult could be seen as a form of child neglect.

Children are aware of body image from an early age, and will usually suffer some degree of playground taunts if they are overweight, so adults should realise that children know if they look different from the crowd. Pretending that these children are perfectly normal will introduce the concept of denial and a false sense of hope that things will somehow change as time goes by. If an unhealthy lifestyle is the cause of an early childhood weight problem and no changes to that lifestyle occur, then the weight problem will continue.

Some families feel that their weight is beyond their control – the whole family are 'big boned' and all have a tendency to be overweight, so the conclusion is that the cause is genetic. Various studies have assessed how much of our size is governed by our genes, and the best estimates are that between 30% and 50% of body size will be under genetic control, but the remaining 50–70% is due to lifestyle.

Of course in any population of people, some are going to be heavier than others and it is one of the joys of the human race that we come in all shapes and sizes. Whilst not wanting to create the impression that everyone should be slim, it is important to recognise that obesity is not simply a cosmetic problem; it causes illness, disability and psychological problems and because it is difficult to treat, prevention is the best approach. Recognising which children would benefit from improving their lifestyle is a vital part of this and parents are in the best position to find this out.

Monitoring a child's growth is discussed in Chapter 3. Body mass index (BMI) may be calculated using the calculator on the website www.healthforallchildren. co.uk and this can be plotted on the BMI chart in Appendix 1 to see if a child's weight is within a healthy range. Alternatively, a family doctor or health visitor can assess this. Ideas for helping an overweight child are discussed in Chapter 10.

In the same way that weight problems may pass unnoticed by family, unhealthy eating patterns can be ignored too. For example, even though a family may realise that there is something wrong with the overall diet (because of a family weight problem), it may be difficult to recognise what aspect of each meal could be improved.

Comments such as 'He has to eat something!', 'A little bit won't hurt' and 'It has milk in it, so it must be good for a child's growth' show how difficult it is to move from an overall viewpoint – 'let's improve the family diet' – to the small print of making each meal a little healthier. The more excuses a family finds to stick to unhealthy eating patterns, the harder it is to tackle the problem, and children will learn to think in the same way. By referring back to *The Balance of Good Health*, detailed in Chapter 1, families can begin to improve the balance of the proportions of daily basic foods to rich foods. Chapter 13 'The Food Frequency Framework' gives more ideas.

Food is used to communicate with children

Many children are happy to eat healthy foods up to a point, but are led astray by well-meaning but uninformed adults. Most adults believe that children prefer junk, and make junk food more highly favoured by using it for treats and rewards and to conveniently relieve hunger between meals. In this way, food is used to communicate success and approval and to alleviate boredom.

Caution is needed if rewarding good behaviour with unhealthy edible treats, because it makes treats more appealing and gives the food a seal of approval by being linked with good behaviour, even if the food is unhealthy. Children will then feel more deprived and reluctant if those foods are discouraged during healthy eating campaigns. It is preferable to make rewards suit the task, so a sporting achievement could merit some new kit, good schoolwork could result in an outing to a science museum or new stationery, and good cookery work could be rewarded by the child taking charge of serving the meal he helped prepare. As children get older, using pocket money as a reward and incentive is good preparation for adulthood, in the same way that salaries motivate the workforce.

Younger kids like burger chain outlets because of the toys and marketing images, not necessarily because the food is that great. But with repeated exposure they develop a liking for the food too. By going along with this, families teach children to be entertained by food, so that it becomes a way of lifting moods, cheering people up and giving a buzz. Whilst on occasion this is not a problem, be wary of ending up with children who can only be entertained when food is on offer (such as kids who feel a trip to the cinema is incomplete without ice-cream and a fizzy drink), who use snacks as the first resort for boredom and who assume that rich foods are a basic ingredient of the daily diet.

Is hunger a reliable trigger for eating?

In prehistoric times, food supply was the major factor that governed survival. Humans evolved as grazing omnivores, meaning that they ate both meat and plant foods whenever they were available. They had to gorge on food in times of plenty to improve their chances of survival when times were hard. However, man would have been discouraged from gorging too much because it would prevent him from running from danger. As man became more adapted, he learned to store food uneaten, rather than store it in his tummy and fat cells, which again improved his survival chances. Hunger was the major stimulus behind his ability to face danger when hunting for food; he didn't face an angry woolly mammoth just for fun.

As man became civilised, the issues that controlled food intake changed dramatically, so that by Victorian times what most people ate was limited by whether they had money to pay for food, sufficient time for food preparation and the seasonal effects on crop harvests. Hunger was a major reason for the necessity of struggling to make ends meet.

Today, in most western societies, cheap food is widely available, often ready prepared so that the minimum of cooking skills are required, and so rich and varied that eating has become a leisure pursuit in itself. Hunger has almost become redundant, and instead, a surrogate marker for boredom. Unless new mechanisms are introduced to control food intake, man will become increasingly prone to gluttony.

Introduce mechanisms to guide food intake and to manage temptation

In addition to encouraging children to tune in to their natural appetite and to pay attention to the sensation of feeling full, other mechanisms can guide children over what and when to eat, remembering that trends learned in childhood will often continue for life.

- *Meal timings and routines*. Whether families eat breakfast is often a household characteristic, but studies show that children concentrate better after eating breakfast and are less likely to snack on unhealthy foods later in the day. Encouraging a good breakfast, a light lunch and a larger tea fits well with a healthy lifestyle, although the main meal of the day may be at lunch-time with a lighter evening meal if food availability is easier this way. If children see this as a normal pattern they will be likely to copy it. However, if parents eat snacks on the hoof, stopping for chips when out shopping regardless of what time of day it is, children will copy this without any clear idea about when chips are appropriate. When unaccompanied as they get older, they will be unaware that chips should form part of a proper meal and that they are unsuitable as a snack between meals.
- *Cost and hassle factors*. Looking at the cost and the amount of preparation a food requires will indicate that some foods are cheap, easy, daily items, but others deserve to be kept for more special days. Now that food is easily available ready prepared, it may be easier to teach children to use the amount of decoration on a food to indicate whether it is a daily basic food or more special. Plain-looking foods, such as a pot of yoghurt, are for weekdays and fancy foods, such as chocolate cheesecake with lashings of whipped cream, are for special occasions. This can help children to feel content rather than deprived when given ordinary foods, even though a fancier item may be in the kitchen cupboard, because they know what to expect.
- *Snack guidance*. Children get used to expecting certain types of food in certain situations. Recently, and encouragingly, moves have been made to promote the eating of fruit as a snack during mid-morning break in UK schools. When everyone does the same with no questions asked, it becomes simply 'the way things are'. Show children that just because chocolates and candy are on sale everywhere, from bookshops to petrol stations, it doesn't mean that it is okay to eat them in each situation. Whether a snack is appropriate has nothing to do with whether a snack is available. If children have never seen parents buy sweets from the supermarket checkout, they will assume that those sweets are simply not for them. But if parents sometimes buy them, children will pester.
- *Household traditions or house rules*. All families have them, although they may call them something different, such as family ways, or customs, or traditions. House rules can be used to teach safety, hygiene and politeness as well as help indecisive children to deal with too much variety. They can help children make healthier choices for themselves and deal with disappointment if the choice was poor.

Are house rules clear to children?

Each household will have a different set of rules: they may be unspoken, and might not appear as a set of rules at all, just comments here and there as situations arise. If the same advice is always given for a particular situation, then that is in effect a house rule. If advice chops and changes according to how parents feel or because they haven't really given the issue much thought, then children will not pick up a clear message.

An area where clear rules can be useful is in how different foods are rated. Rating foods as daily basics, weekend foods or rare treats is a method for knowing how often richer foods can be safely enjoyed. This is covered in more detail in Chapter 13.

Other ways of teaching children about eating appropriately may be to talk about the cost, the ease of preparation, seasonal factors such as why we do not usually eat strawberries at Christmas, and whether a food is to hand. For example, if a requested food is not in the cupboard on a Sunday evening, then it won't be possible to get hold of it, however upset the child may be. If the child learns to understand that an empty cupboard means 'no chance', then it may save distress to both child and parent.

As children try more variety they will get an idea of likes and dislikes, so when faced with a huge choice, they can be reminded of their own tendencies. For example, if a child doesn't like nuts then avoid sweets or ice-cream with nuts in.

When thinking about house rules, try to make positive rules rather than negative ones. Children accept guidance on what they *can* do far more easily than rules about what is forbidden. Box 9.1 contains ideas for making house rules positive.

Box 9.1 Making house rules positive rather than negative

Negative house rules

- No more eating after cleaning teeth before bed.
- No more than half your pocket money to be spent on edible things.
- Junk food is not allowed in the half hour leading up to a meal.
- Sticky things are not to be eaten on the sofa.
- Do not keep eating once you feel full.
- Do not run with a lolly stick in your mouth.
- Do not leave muddy footprints indoors.
- Children do not get if they do not say please and thank you.
- Do not pretend breakages are not your fault – ask an adult to help clear up the mess.
- Do not moan if you do not like what you chose.
- Crisps are not an essential part of a packed lunch.
- Just because children are hungry doesn't mean that they need to eat.
- Do not eat if not feeling hungry.

Positive house rules

- Make toothpaste the last thing you taste each night.
- At least half of pocket money to be saved or spent on things to treasure.

- Fruit is allowed in the half hour leading up to a meal.
- Sticky things are to be eaten in a place that is easy to clean up.
- If you feel full, stop eating.
- Take things out of your mouth before running, in case you trip.
- Muddy shoes are to be left outside.
- Good manners are the norm, not a rare display for grandparents.
- If glass or china gets broken, inform an adult rather than hide the evidence.
- When trying a new food, ask to try a little bit first in case you do not like it.
- Packed lunches contain sandwiches and fruit, plus a few extras that sometimes include crisps.
- It is good to feel hungry in the time leading up to a meal. Use 'safe snacks' or distraction from hunger when a meal is not due.
- Eating when not hungry puts people at risk of eating too much.

Tailor house rules to suit both parents and children. After all, they are there to make life easier for everyone, not to complicate things.

Summary points

- Children sense when parents are lacking in confidence and may then test confidence in other areas. Parents can use incentives to show children that they are in control.
- Children need to practise making decisions whilst parents are around to guide the process. If all their decisions are made for them then they may grow up to be either timid and lacking in self-confidence or determined to try out everything that was forbidden in childhood.
- Ignoring weight problems in children is unhelpful in the long run. There are lots of positive ways to help a child put health on the priority list without causing distress or worsening self-esteem.
- Make sure that food is not used to communicate unhealthy messages to children and that junk food does not become central to how children like to be entertained.
- Because hunger is no longer a reliable trigger for eating, introduce mechanisms that guide when and what to eat and help to manage temptation.
- Use positive house rules to help children feel good about what they *can* do, rather than irritated about what they shouldn't.

Chapter 10

Helping an overweight child

For a junior-aged child who is already overweight, progress will require working out what factors lie behind the weight problem. Forcing a healthy diet will be unsuccessful, whereas finding positive solutions to troublesome eating patterns or a dislike of exercise will produce welcome improvements.

Recognise problems as early as possible, preferably before they start at all

Better pay the cook than the doctor!

This saying sums up a useful approach to life – prevention is better than cure. By living healthily from the start, there will be less need for cures. There is plenty of evidence to show that heart disease, diabetes and many types of cancer are less common if the diet is good, as outlined in Chapter 12.

Being overweight in childhood is not something to brush aside with an 'Oh, he'll grow out of it' comment. Weight problems in children are strongly coupled with psychological problems and low self-esteem, as well as heart disease and diabetes in later life. Even if an overweight child achieves normal weight in adulthood, they still carry a higher risk of the latter conditions than if weight had always been normal. Learning to overeat and to be inactive during childhood will also increase the likelihood of continuing the same lifestyle in adulthood. Children will benefit tremendously from guidance about being healthy, and this includes recognising problems when they are there.

As already mentioned in Chapter 9, the Earlybird study showed that parents are not good at recognising when children carry too much weight – an alarming percentage of parents described their children as 'about right' when they were not (*see* page 103). However, this does not mean that children should be labelled with terms that will merely get them down and be upsetting, as this will be both hurtful and counter-productive. Instead, look for ways to help children become interested in being healthy and keeping fit, and give extra help to those children who need it most.

Parents should aim to keep a rough idea about their child's build in mind – do not guess, check it out from time to time. The growth charts in a child's health record (the red book in the UK) are for 0 to 18 years of age. Plot a child's height and weight to see if they still follow the same centile lines as in earlier childhood. If weight has crept across more than one centile line, or if height and weight are following very different lines (such as one on the 25th centile and the other on the 75th), then discuss with the family doctor about calculating body mass index, which will give a more accurate idea about whether weight is appropriate for

Table 10.1 Average changes that occur during puberty

	Age of growth spurt onset	*Change in body tissue*	*Average annual weight gain*	*Average annual height increase*
Before puberty			2.5 kg	5 cm
Girls	10–13 years	Gain lean tissue and fat	5 kg	6 cm
Boys	12–15 years	Gain lean tissue and lose fat	6 kg	7 cm

height and age. Alternatively, this can be calculated using an online BMI calculator, such as at www.healthforallchildren.co.uk on the parent's page.

Understand about normal growth spurts

Many parents feel relaxed about their child's size because of the simple fact that it keeps changing. Children grow in fits and starts and their appetites vary accordingly, so parents may notice that a slim phase is followed by a chubby phase and then a growth spurt. This is normal. However, be cautious about attributing prolonged chubbiness to a forthcoming growth spurt because it may signal that the child is carrying more weight than the growth spurt will use up, so that chubbiness persists.

It is healthy for children to store some fat in preparation for the rapid growth that accompanies puberty. Table 10.1 shows average changes that occur during puberty. The growth spurt usually lasts about three years, but some children grow more quickly over a shorter time and others may grow more slowly for longer.

A child's appetite will increase to match periods of rapid growth. Calcium is an important part of the diet to ensure good bone formation and is found in dairy products, cereals and green vegetables. Parents should watch that they do not continue to push extra-sized helpings at the end of a growth spurt when appetite usually tails off, or children will eat too much. Always try to tune in to a child's natural appetite.

Children require the same food balance during periods of rapid growth as they do at other times, even if more food is eaten. Changing the balance to include more junk foods or sugary snacks will increase the risk of obesity and may push healthier foods off the menu so that essential nutrients are in short supply. Instead, keep the proportions of fruit and vegetables, carbohydrates and proteins as before, but increase their portion sizes to match appetite. A child can safely eat masses of fruit and vegetables to stem hunger without upsetting the overall balance of the diet.

Dieting is inappropriate for children

Even if a child falls into the overweight or obese category, it will not be helpful to put a child 'on a diet'. In very basic terms, a diet can be seen as 'a restricted way of eating with the aim of weight reduction'. Neither restricting a child's diet nor aiming for weight reduction is appropriate for a growing child. By looking to stabilise weight and promote healthy eating habits, they should 'grow into their weight' as growth in height continues. Losing weight should not be necessary and may mean a shortage of nutrients for healthy growth. If the rate of weight gain slows down, the child will gradually reach a stage when weight is more appropriate for height (*see* Figure 10.1).

An example of weight stabilisation

The growth charts in Figure 10.1 show how a child who has gone through an obese phase (as shown during the years 8 to 10) can stabilise weight by slowing down the rate of weight gain rather than actually losing weight. In this way, even though weight still increases with each year, it gradually becomes more appropriate for the child's height. See how the BMI actually falls, even though weight has continued to slowly increase. By the end of the teenage growth spurt, height and weight both fall into a healthy range without weight loss having occurred at any stage.

Instead of restricting the diet by counting calories or banning certain foods, aim to encourage all the healthy ingredients whilst taking away the focus of food as entertainment and comfort, so reducing the desire for too much junk food.

The negative effects of dieting are discussed further in the companion book *Weight Matters for Young People*.

Fitness is the key to good health

People come in all shapes and sizes and it would be untrue to suggest that only overweight people are prone to illness. For example, a slim but unfit person may carry an increased risk of heart disease just as much as a fitter but heavier person. It is reassuring that even if weight remains high, the chance of illness can be reduced by getting fitter. In order for exercise to improve health, it does not necessarily have to bring about weight reduction.

If one looks at the BMI of a fine sportsman such as Sir Matthew Pinsent during his phenomenal rowing career, it would appear that he was overweight. (At around 16 stone, 8 lbs and a height of 6'5", his BMI was around 27.6, which falls into the overweight range.) But his excess weight was mainly muscle and his heart should be in great shape due to his high level of exercise.

Some of the benefits of staying fit include:

- Exercise converts excess fat into muscle.
- Fitness keeps blood vessels cleaner and exercises the heart.
- Exercise improves the types of fat that are carried in the blood, such as cholesterol level.
- Exercise increases bone strength and keeps joints supple.
- Exercise can broaden people's enjoyment of things and create more ideas for having fun.
- Exercise can have a very powerful effect on the way people value themselves and on their self-esteem.

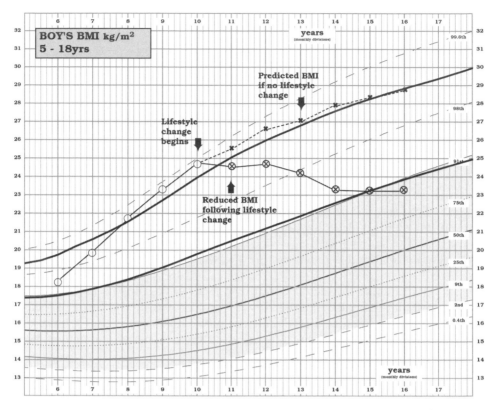

Figure 10.1 BMI growth charts. Reproduced by kind permission of the Child Growth Foundation. The two thick lines on the chart represent the International Obesity Task Force definitions for obesity (upper) and overweight (lower).

- People can enjoy eating richer foods if they use up plenty of energy by exercising.
- People enjoy a sense of achievement and of team spirit when they have attained goals or enjoyed a match.

It is important to emphasise how it is good to get fit for the sake of fitness, rather than as a way of reducing weight. If people see exercise only as a way of reducing weight then their motivation will be weaker than if they appreciate the wide variety of benefits it brings.

Remember that life is a long journey – there is no need to get the whole thing perfect in one go. Teach principles that will help children through the ups and downs of life, to increase the chance that as body shape fluctuates it will vary within a healthy range.

Which factors have led to the child's weight problem?

In a family where one or several members are overweight, there will usually be more than one reason behind it. Discovering which issues apply will lead to varied strategies for improving the whole household's health. Even if only one child appears overweight, the best approach will be to look at family eating and

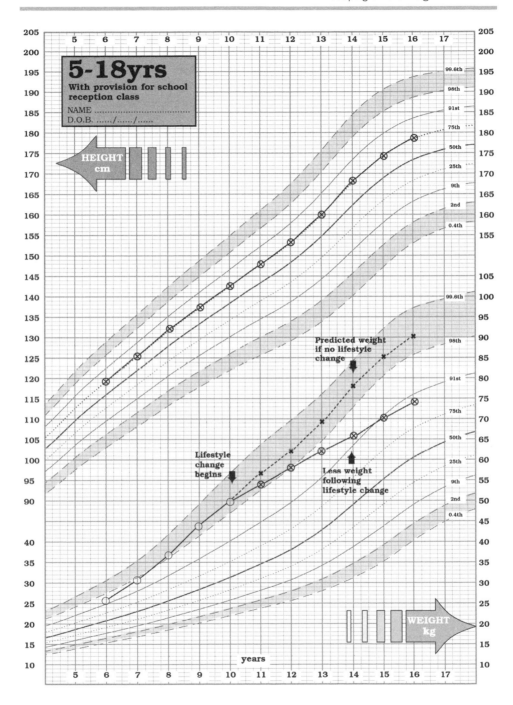

exercise patterns in general. Picking on one person and giving special treatment is a way of worsening their body image and reducing confidence, so creating more of an uphill struggle.

Additionally, if one member of the family is carrying too much weight, then it may indicate that others will eventually follow suit because health and fitness have not been a family priority.

Which of the following factors apply?

- Comfort eating? Has low self-esteem or sadness led to comfort eating? Have parents tried to cheer up their child with food?
- Is the child always hungry with what seems to be an unnaturally big appetite?
- Have family behaviour patterns led a child to clear the plate and eat whatever is provided?
- Has the family chosen whatever seems tasty and popular, whilst giving little thought to nutrition, weight or fitness?

Comfort eating

When life is tough, food can be one of the reliable ways of finding pleasure and relief. For some people in very difficult situations, food may be the only joy on the horizon. Furthermore, people need to eat, but it is rarely obvious whether a particular mouthful is a necessity or whether it just tastes nice. It is easy to slip into the habit of eating when feeling down, whilst using the excuse that it is because it is needed.

Indeed, if people get used to a diet high in sugary foods they may go on to develop sugar cravings, making them feel light-headed and shaky. The obvious treatment seems to be more sugar, so that a sugary snack then seems perfectly justifiable. This triggers a vicious circle of feeling both physically and mentally better by eating, although in reality this well-being is usually short-lived. If a person is prone to sugar cravings it is preferable to eat starchy foods rather than sugary ones, such as a piece of toast, which will be released slowly into the bloodstream, so that further surges of blood sugar are avoided.

Children may make the discovery of cheering themselves up by eating rich foods, but more often it is taught by friends and family. From an early age we stop tears with treats and we comfort with sweets. It can become difficult to separate the giving of food from showing love for children. If a mother has found herself in this position, of showing her affection by providing delicious home cooking or a ready supply of treats, then she may feel that a health drive would require rejecting and neglecting her children. A child, too, might feel rejected if this is the way they feel assured of their parent's love. Hence health drives must be discussed and agreed upon, with clear and positive reasons for change and good communication to avoid feelings of rejection.

Some children learn to gain popularity by giving food – or 'status snacks' – to friends. A child in the playground who hands out toffees and crisps to anyone that will be friends will become popular, although it would be a harsh lesson to then find popularity fading if the food supply dries up. Usually children have a naturally self-centred core, so to be able to freely hand out sweets to others suggests either an inborn generosity of spirit – in which case, such a child will be popular throughout life – or that the child is so well provided with sweets that they can be safely shared because there are still plenty for later.

Action points include:

- Be clear about how children are shown that they are loved and valued. Conveying this through food creates problems, so use lots of other ways to show feelings, such as by giving attention and using words not food. Meals can be made special regardless of what is on the menu (*see* Box 10.1 for ideas).

- Avoid short-term food solutions for low moods. Resorting to rich snacks creates problems in the long run, even if it helps in the short term. Teach children to talk about their feelings rather than suppress them with food, and build on healthy eating patterns alongside ways to boost self-esteem so that the need for comfort foods is less.
- Avoid dosing up with more simple sugars during a sugar crave. Encourage children to eat complex carbohydrates, starchy foods or a portion of fruit instead, as these foods won't cause the rapid rise and fall in blood sugar that sugary things will.
- Talk to children about how and why people value their friends. People do not necessarily like the ones with the most money, the best clothes or the biggest house – it is personality that counts. A friendship means caring and sharing the same sense of humour and interests, rather than sharing food. Whilst generosity is a wonderful thing, make sure children understand that some-times people can be used if they appear too willing to share.

Box 10.1 Ideas for making ordinary meals special

- Sit down as a family whenever possible – do not let the television take over mealtime conversation and attention.
- Choose mealtime themes or variety night ideas, as suggested in Chapter 13.
- Use candles or unusual table decorations.
- Use unusual implements, such as chopsticks, a fondue set or kebab skewers.
- Invite friends around for a meal.
- Eat in unusual settings, such as outside or picnics in the car.
- Plan some topics to discuss before sitting down, such as holiday plans, new jokes or birthday party plans, so that the food on offer will not be the main focus of the meal.
- Avoid topics that may generate upset, such as progress at school or bedroom tidiness.
- Include children in adult conversation. Bored children will either overeat or misbehave in an attempt to entertain themselves.

Coping with a large appetite

In any population some people will be larger than others and some smaller than the rest. Unfortunately, too many people now fall into the larger end of the scale because modern lifestyles make it hard to get the correct balance between energy in (eating) and energy out (exercise). A large appetite will need to be accompan-ied by high levels of activity or it will lead to obesity. Chapter 11 looks at ways to boost exercise and activity in junior-aged children. The next section looks at ways to contain an overenthusiastic appetite.

Being bored is not the same as feeling hungry

If a child is fairly active but tucks into too much rich food, it is worth checking whether they are eating out of boredom. Food has become part of the entertainment culture and with its ready availability on every corner and in every situation, it is easy to use it to liven up dull moments, to fill the gap between activities and to take away the tedium of boring stretches, such as a long journey.

Challenge children about how hungry they really are and look at the healthy body jigsaw together (*see* Chapter 8) to make health relevant. Show how the balance of food intake over the whole day could be improved by choosing healthier snacks and by getting busy in order to relieve boredom. Watch out for fizzy drinks, which can add many calories into the diet without filling up a child. *See* Chapter 13 for more information on healthy snacks and drinks.

Car journeys can be enlivened with car games, story tapes and music. Store up family topics to discuss in the car, such as planning out DIY projects or what equipment will be needed for the next holiday. Some families might even find a relaxing, tranquil silence will make a change. If food is appropriate, think of it in terms of the overall day's nutrition rather than as an extra, and take the opportunity to hand out fresh or dried fruit, plain crackers or breadsticks, which may go down well if nothing else is available, so helping children to develop a taste for healthier snacks.

Suggest that children fill the gaps between activities with either nutritious foods or by chewing gum or liquorice root, or by getting busy with another activity.

For those dull moments in life it is vital that children find ways of coping without having to eat. If children eat snacks whenever they are bored, their health will suffer and their dentists will be busy! By helping children tune in to the difference between boredom and hunger they will hopefully begin to judge what they eat and why.

Teach children not to fear being hungry

With endless claims that bizarre diets will help weight loss without ever having to feel hungry, anyone would think that this sensation is dangerous. A useful guide to healthy eating is that if people do not feel slightly hungry before each meal then they are probably eating too much or too often.

Hunger is a useful sensation but it can be allowed to take over. Because young children are prone to getting fractious when hungry – and that means noise and hassle for parents – the tendency is to feed children sooner rather than later, so that their behaviour doesn't deteriorate into a full-blown tantrum. As children grow, they must learn to tolerate hunger because life isn't always organised and a meal isn't always ready or appropriate. Also, because growth happens in fits and starts, a filling meal one day may be insufficient in the midst of a growth spurt and it may take a few hungry afternoons before the child adjusts mealtime intake.

Teach children to cope with feeling hungry between meals by using distraction, such as getting busy, and by encouraging them to feel pleased that hunger means the next meal will be enjoyed all the more. Use house rules to get children used to the idea of not eating rich snacks in the time leading up to a meal.

Improve the balance of a child's diet so that eating large amounts will not matter so much

Using *The Balance of Good Health* (*see* Chapter 1), parents can learn to increase the healthy ingredients on a plate, whilst reducing the portion sizes of high-fat items such as pies and full-fat dairy products. This will lower the energy density of the meal, so that for the same number of mouthfuls, the child will run less risk of eating more calories than are needed. Children should be encouraged to eat as much fruit and vegetables as they wish and to use starchy foods such as rice, bread or pasta (complex carbohydrates) to fill up on rather than high-fat or sugary items. Moving to lower-fat meals means that eating large amounts is less of a problem. Ideas to help children enjoy fresh produce are given in Chapter 12.

Use household routines to introduce healthy eating and double-check that existing rules are not encouraging bad habits

Chapter 1 looked at how household traditions can override a child's natural appetite, so that children learn to ignore their own fullness signals and be guided by parents' wishes or house rules instead. The commonest examples are of children being encouraged to clear their plate and for pudding to be used as a reward for eating the first course. If families have used these approaches then they should discuss changes together, because it is important for all the family to understand why things are to change. In particular, both parents must try to give the same messages to children or chaos will result.

Action points include:

- Put children in charge of portion sizes, whilst encouraging smaller portions in general and giving the option of a second helping if still hungry. Encourage variety by putting small amounts of new things on the plate.
- Try to slow down the process of eating, so that the sensation of fullness has time to kick in during the meal. Fullness signals take a few minutes to trigger, so a very rapid meal may not give that bloated feeling until several minutes after ceasing to eat. By slowing down the process of eating, a child can learn to tune in to this sensation to guide when enough has been eaten. Encourage children to chew food properly and to take smaller mouthfuls. Make conversation during meals. Serving fiddly foods such as corn on the cob and food that is assembled on the plate, such as fajitas, is another way to slow down the eating process.
- Use starters as a way of drawing out the length of the meal and of promoting healthy items. Offer slices of melon, a bowl of salad or some chopped raw vegetables as a starter when children are most hungry, which will increase the chance of them being eaten, rather than offering them at the end of a meal when they are already full.
- Ask children halfway through a meal whether they are nearly full. If they are not used to thinking about this then a timely reminder may help them tune in.
- Tell children what is for pudding so they can reserve some room. If the pudding forms part of a balanced diet there is no need to use it as a reward or to forbid it if insufficient food was eaten during the first course.
- If a child feels starving in the half hour before a meal is ready, either think of an easy starter or suggest that they eat pudding before the main course. There is no great reason why puddings must follow main courses: this will not 'spoil an appetite' because the child is still being offered the meal that was planned – just in a different order. At the end of a meal, remind children to tune in to whether they are still hungry before offering second helpings.

- Be confident that children *can* make good choices when given the opportunity. Many parents fear that their children will not know how to choose appropriately (e.g. meal size, amount of sweets eaten, etc.) and so tell their children what and when to eat, thinking that is best. But childhood is about letting children find things out whilst parental guidance is available. If children do not have a go then they will never learn. Let them make their own mistakes, but discuss the outcome together so they have the opportunity to learn. Congratulate good choices too.

Do children manipulate treat foods in exchange for good behaviour?

From early childhood, many parents use food as a way of rewarding good behaviour, so it is not surprising that some children learn the same tactic – to reward parents with good behaviour in exchange for food. Who is in control in the household? Whilst one of the aims of this book is to allow children to take control over their own eating, this should not be confused with allowing children to control other people by the way that they eat.

If a child has slipped into a pattern of bad temper and misery unless favourite foods are on offer, it will take a while to move out of this phase. Begin by encouraging a broader variety of foods, perhaps by including small portions of new things in addition to favourite foods, and then gradually reduce portion sizes of the favourites. In this way the overall balance will improve whilst introducing new foods, but without having to forego the things a child wants. Children can become experts at detecting a parent's anxiety triggers; therefore if mealtime battles are common, introduce change gradually and quietly so they have little to react against at any one meal.

Be very clear about the difference between a child who likes specific foods and one who just likes to get their own way. Remember that most children will respond to all manner of inducements to behave, such as stickers for young children, whereas pocket money or being excused from household chores become far more useful negotiating tools for older children. Reassure them that limiting the frequency of unhealthy foods is not a sign of disapproval of their behaviour, but a sign that they are worth caring about.

How important has nutrition and fitness been to the family?

In the average busy household there are numerous things to worry about, so it is no wonder that nutrition is not high on everyone's list. However, by ignoring the warning signs we do children no favours at all.

Weight, as any overweight adult will know, can be very difficult to lose. It is easier to keep it off in the first place than to gain too much and then face the struggle of losing it. Allowing children to become overweight means they are being given another problem to either sort out or live with, and living with a weight problem is not much fun. In addition, if they are encouraged to think of themselves as fine when they are not, they are learning a form of denial. Whilst children should have self-belief and feel proud of themselves, false reassurance can be very confusing. This becomes more significant as children go through puberty when self-esteem becomes much more entangled with body image.

Denying problems, especially if a child has become aware of body image due to teasing at school, means not having to deal with them, but those problems will still be there the next day and the day after and the day after that. Passing off chubbiness as acceptable puppy fat and continuing an unhealthy lifestyle means that a child will learn denial – when parents ignore weight problems children do so too.

Where possible, children should be helped to look positively at the things that can be tackled, such as getting fitter and improving the balance of the diet, without focusing particularly on body shape or weight. Small improvements to lifestyle that continue throughout childhood and into adulthood will be worth a huge amount in the end, particularly as small changes are more achievable. More goals can always be added in if things go well. If first attempts to boost lifestyle fall flat, back off for a short while and then start again, perhaps trying a different tack.

Making excuses is a form of denial

It is natural for parents to feel protective of their children and to try to make them happy. But parents should be cautious about attributing problems to unlikely causes and be realistic about excuses. Less than 5% of overweight children have an underlying illness or condition that causes being overweight. Whilst there are some uncommon genetic, congenital or endocrine conditions that cause obesity, as a general rule these will be associated with short stature and sometimes other abnormalities. Parents should speak to their family doctor if there are concerns about the chance of an underlying condition.

The great majority (95%) of people who are overweight have an imbalance of how much they eat compared to how much energy they use up. Making an excuse for a child's large appetite or lack of interest in sports is a way of avoiding doing anything about it. As a general rule, excuses are a barrier to change and are unhelpful.

Things do not have to change all in one go. Start with easy targets that parent and child feel they can achieve, and then plan to build on these. If parents feel tempted to make excuses and continue old eating and inactivity patterns, they should talk to their child about how they feel as a parent. Surprisingly, the motivation to improve things will sometimes come not from parents but from their child. School projects will often strike a chord with children, so take advantage of school initiatives that extol the benefits of drinking water or promote eating fruit or walking to school. Pick up leaflets, share tips with friends, try new ideas. Put health somewhere on the family priority list.

Summary points

- Prevention is better than cure. Keep an eye on a child's growth so that unhealthy tendencies can be picked up early on when change is easier.
- Growing (and hence hungry) children need the same balance of foods as ever, rather than free access to junk food. Remind children to tune in to hunger, especially at the end of a growth spurt when appetite tails off.
- Improving fitness will improve health regardless of whether weight changes.
- Instead of using food to comfort or cheer children up, explore other ways to show how much they are valued.
- Teach children to be able to tolerate feeling hungry and to recognise whether they are feeling hungry or just bored.
- Slow meals down so that 'fullness cues' have more chance to kick in and guide how much is eaten.
- Reduce the chance of being manipulated over food by avoiding its use as a reward.
- Put nutrition and fitness firmly onto the family priority list.

Chapter 11

Kids will be active if they can

Because modern lifestyles use up less energy for daily activities (due to changes in transport, central heating, entertainment and fewer manual jobs than in years gone by), children need to find ways to actively boost exercise in order to avoid health problems. This chapter looks at ways to lift barriers and encourage motivation to exercise.

Are children doing enough exercise at present?

Put simply, no. Only a third of girls and just over half of boys get the recommended amount of physical activity of one hour per day. This is not just because of computer games and television, but reflects changes in society. Children cycle less than in the past, partly due to safety fears but also to inconveniences such as regulations about children needing to be accompanied when attending clubs. They walk less, which reflects the increase in car travel, plus they can get in touch with friends by using mobile phones and email and without having to leave the house. Towns have changed, with more distant or isolated housing estates and out-of-town shopping malls meaning fewer young-sters wander down to town to meet with friends or walk with family to the shops. Car travel continues to increase with cars becoming affordable to more of the population. The media have become hugely powerful in bringing news and messages about 'stranger danger' and child safety into our homes, with the result that parents are fearful of allowing children out alone. These and many other factors have led children to stay indoors more and get used to a sedentary life, because getting exercise now involves effort and organisation.

Parents can check to see if their own children are getting enough exercise by answering the Child Activity Assessment questions listed in Box 3.1 in Chapter 3. They will give a good idea about whether or not a child is active enough. Another way to assess activity is to take a look at the things a child likes doing after school and at weekends. If children prefer quiet games, watching TV, colouring and reading, for example, or perhaps computer games, jigsaws and watching motor sport videos, then it may be that they are not getting enough exercise for good health. If the toys in the garden are hardly used, a child's slippers are far tattier than their trainers and the suggestion of a walk in the park is met with a hostile rant, then parents should feel confident that tackling this area can only be a good thing!

For determined couch potatoes, the 'right' amount of exercise is anything more than they are doing now, but the first aim is to increase the enjoyment from more active pastimes so they will be more popular in future.

Incorporate the following action points whenever possible, aiming to achieve them on at least five days each week:

- Encourage children to get out of breath from some activity most days.
- Aim to get about an hour of exercise in total throughout the day – made up of several shorter bursts or a long stretch if preferred.
- Ask children how much exercise they have had that day. If they do not even think about it, they won't make any effort.
- Agree a daily television and computer game time limit. Help children both to monitor this and think of it as a positive improvement rather than a ban.

Setting good activity ground rules – which mean ordinary habits that the family follow without question – is very helpful, particularly as it can help children to keep up some exercise as they go through the teenage years, when activity levels tend to reduce significantly. Examples might be going for a Sunday walk, aiming for a weekly swim or hiring bikes when on holiday. Cutting down on television, whatever a child does instead, has been shown to improve health.

What approaches help to get kids off the sofa?

The following sections explore two different approaches to this question. The first is to overcome practical barriers to exercise, which include physical and time barriers, neighbourhood issues and unhelpful household routines. The second approach is to overcome a child's lack of interest in getting fit, including assessing confidence, self-esteem and emotional problems that can have a big impact on activity.

Practical barriers to exercise

If people do not value keeping fit, then they will not do so. A frequent response in my surgery, when people are asked how much exercise they get, is 'I haven't got time'. This isn't actually an answer to the question, but it reveals a lot about the person because it shows that whilst being busy, they are aware of an unhealthy lifestyle and feel guilty about not doing more to prioritise health. It is obvious when a person does value exercise because the response is quite different: 'Well I usually try to do this sport or that activity, but I struggle to fit everything in sometimes.'

It is likely that both groups – the keen ones and the unenthusiastic – are equally tied up with work and family commitments. The difference between them is their interest and enthusiasm for a healthy lifestyle rather than any major difference in free time, because it reflects how people like to spend their free time. Children will learn to manage their timetables and prioritise their activities by copying parents – busy parents often have busy children; laid-back parents often have children who are easygoing. If parents can't find time for keeping fit, then this will rub off on the family. Active parents are far more likely to end up with active kids.

Parents can show that they value activities within a busy schedule

Whilst it would be lovely for everyone to pop along to the squash court twice a week and fit in a round of golf each Sunday, life simply isn't like that. However, adults can show children that fitness is important even if they struggle to do much themselves.

Action points include:

- Grab time whenever possible. There is no need to set aside two hours for a full match and warm-up exercises are not essential. Just do a bit here and there, even if it's only five minutes jogging up the street or round the garden before getting on with the chores. The shorter the bursts, the more likely kids might join in too.
- Be active even when not exercising. Run up the stairs, dance around the house and consider parking the car further away and enjoying a brisk walk.
- Do not bother with kit. If the opportunity arises to kick a ball, join in a race or paddle a canoe, do not be put off by the wrong shoes or too smart an outfit – just join in.
- Which is more important? A tidy house or a healthy heart? Think about priorities – could household chores be pruned or delegated to create a little more time for fitness?
- Do not worry about freshness either. If jogging in the 20 minutes before work means arriving feeling hot and bothered, just roll on some deodorant and do not give it another thought. Many people die from lack of exercise, but I've yet to hear of anyone dying from sweaty armpits!

Show that children's activities are valued too

Even if parents have trouble exercising themselves, whether due to timetable problems or perhaps because of a disability, exercise can still be an important theme.

Action points include:

- Know what team games and sports a child is doing at school. Ask about what position the child plays, who the good players are and what the PE teacher is like. Get to know the rules so that everyone can share in discussions about foul play, impressive tackles and how to improve tactics.
- Check up on what kit is needed. Particularly if a child is sensitive or prone to being picked on, having the wrong kit can have disastrous effects on confidence in taking part.
- Help children to remember what kit is needed on which day. Some kids are great at this but others are simply hopeless. Do not let a disorganised personality be the cause of missing games or swimming.
- Be prepared to take children to clubs and team practice after school, and help them to get to know other children there by getting to know other parents. Children will enjoy sports all the more if they feel they are meeting up with friends.
- Wherever possible, resist excuses to miss games. Children who hate PE might find any number of ways to miss it. Try not to collude with a child by going along with fictitious headaches or magic tummy ache – the one that vanishes 15 minutes after games are over.
- If children really hate team sports, show enthusiasm for other activities such as Scouts or Brownies, walking a dog (even if it needs to be 'borrowed' from a neighbour), or helpful tasks such as leaf sweeping in the autumn and washing the car.

Does the neighbourhood help or hinder activities?

Alongside increased car use and the reduction in walking and cycling, there is now less tolerance of noisy kids playing in the street and a much greater emphasis on child safety. Many parents, particularly if they do not have a garden or if they are surrounded by communal grounds, feel reluctant to let children play outside unaccompanied. Some families have grumbling neighbours who won't tolerate footballs coming over the wall or the normal racket that comes from children having fun, thus parents feel pressured to keep kids quiet rather than busy. It can help to talk to other neighbours who have similar aged children. Is it possible to set up a supervision rota for outdoor play? Do nearby friends have a garden for play on dry days and who can come round for indoor play when it is raining or dark? Children are more easily entertained when there are friends to play with, which can help if putting limits on television time. Box 11.1 gives suggestions for opportunities for activity.

As children get older, they can be allowed short spells of unsupervised play outside as long as they have learned about safety, i.e. not to talk to strangers, not to go on main roads and the boundaries of how far from the door they can go. Parents might find out about doing cycling proficiency; lending a child a mobile phone if going slightly further afield and explaining which strangers are safe to approach in an emergency.

Box 11.1 Opportunities for activity

- Most schools allow children to be dropped off at least ten minutes before the bell rings. If a child likes charging around the playground with other early friends, this can add almost an hour of extra activity each week.
- Some supermarkets and big stores have a crèche or ball play area that will entertain a child whilst parents get on with the shopping.
- An organisational approach might help. For example, plan a regular stop-off at the park each Wednesday.
- Send children along with an outdoor toy when they are invited out for tea.
- Consider leaving a fold-up scooter, football, skipping rope or roller skates in the boot of the car so that kids can make the most of chances when out and about.

Dropping children further away from school is becoming popular, and has been formalised by some schools into 'walking bus' schemes: a few parents arrange to meet at specified places on the way to school, collecting children as they walk along. Everyone gets a healthy start to the day, and parking pressure around the school is eased greatly. Some local authorities have been very supportive, helping with clear signposts to warn motorists and luminous jackets to keep the children safe. Do any local schools have such a scheme? Could parents join up with a few others on a smaller scale to set up an informal version of a walking bus? Schools might be happy to look into it if parents brought it to their attention. Further details are available on the Walking Bus website www.walkingbus.com. Even if there is no formal scheme, families could fit a walk into their timetable by setting off a little earlier and parking further away.

Develop a 'play in the garden' zone

Parents can encourage children to play safely outdoors by creating a 'play zone' in the garden. Some large toys can be hired from the local toy library, available through the local council, and swapped from time to time to reduce the chance of children getting bored. Club together with grandparents to buy a large toy, such as a climbing frame or trampoline (*see* Box 11.2), for a special birthday present. Further swings or a slide can be added to modular climbing frames at later intervals. Keep an eye on the local paper for bargains or consider advertising for second-hand equipment if it can be checked that it is in good order.

More ideas are available at www.playday.org.uk and information relating to safe play is available through the Royal Society for the Prevention of Accidents at www.rospa.co.uk/playsafety.

Box 11.2 Trampoline safety advice

- Place well away from trees, walls or fences.
- Clear objects away from the surrounding ground.
- Use a frame pad to cover the spring system.
- Remind children to remove restricting clothing or items that could get caught, such as scarves.
- Only one person should use the trampoline at any one time.
- Do not allow children to bounce from the trampoline onto other surfaces.

Build up confidence and interest in taking part

Teach skills and practise games together

The great thing about practice is that little and often is just as good as long spells at a game. Most parents can find the odd five minutes to join in with something, so there is no need to be put off by having to find half an hour to help a child with sports. Find a couple of minutes here and there to kick or catch a ball, do some running together or cycle around the block. The more practice a child has out of school, the more their confidence will build in taking part at school. Improving general fitness will help a child cope with many aspects of life, not just PE. A parent's involvement will make exercise seem important, help boost general confidence and also add to the daily quota of exercise.

Incentives can be used to get a child involved. One incentive is to generate some competition and another is to use rewards.

Be competitive

Whilst taking care not to put off a reluctant child even more, explore competing safely with a parent as a way of building up the competitive spirit. Short spells with an easy goal are a good way to start, such as 'beat you to the post box' or 'see who can skip the longest without stopping'. 'Bet you can't!' is another phrase that many children respond to. Make sure that children are not allowed to win every time, because this will soon be noticed and may leave the child feeling belittled.

If parent and child are starting a new regular activity together, both could try a little experiment. At the start, run up and down the stairs as fast as possible, counting how many trips are made before feeling exhausted. Repeat this some weeks later to see how much fitness has improved. Stair running could be used as a daily activity in itself, particularly in the winter, and it is great to see how quickly the scores improve. Post scores on the fridge and challenge other family members to do better!

Alternatively, try a 'Catch 10' competition. All that is needed is a bouncy ball and a brick wall. See who can get furthest without dropping the ball:

> Throw against the wall. (Once)
> Throw and clap twice before catching. (Twice)
> Hit the ground then up to the wall then catch. (Three times, etc.)
> Throw from behind your back.
> Throw under your leg.
> Throw, turn around, then catch.
> Throw with the right and catch with the left hand.
> Throw with the left and catch with the right hand.
> Throw, touch the ground and catch.
> Throw with your eyes shut and catch.

Use rewards that suit the achievement

There are plenty of non-food ways to reward success and effort. Pocket money is one option, or earning kit and sports equipment can be very motivating. If a child is starting a new sport or club, try to beg or borrow the required equipment to begin with, partly so that the child will not feel guilty if enthusiasm wanes and the whole thing is a disaster, but also so that looking forward to purchasing the right gear or sport accessories can be a worthwhile goal in itself.

Because using food as a reward makes it seem special and can make children fond of unhealthy treats, try to avoid using rich or sugary foods to celebrate achievements. Be aware that handing out a standard confectionery bar or slab of chocolate at the end of a game of sports may mean that more calories are eaten than were used up throughout the game (see Table 11.1).

Wherever possible, remember that food should be seen as nutrition rather than as a reward. If the chosen snack is considered a reasonable part of the overall diet,

Table 11.1 Comparison of number of calories used up in various exercise activities with number of calories contained in some popular snacks

Activity (minutes)	Calories used up	Snack (grams)	Calories contained
Moderate cycling (30)	100	Mars bar (62.5)	281
Moderate running (20)	148	Kit Kat chunky (55)	290
Swimming (30)	130	Snickers (64.5)	323
Table tennis (30)	160	Packet of crisps (34.5)	181
Golf (60)	160	Lucozade energy original drink (380 ml)	277

then fine, but if it is in addition to nutritious meals then be aware that some snacks and sugary drinks can add an awful lot of calories with very little useful nutrition.

In particular, avoid the routine of providing chocolate or crisps automatically following any game of sports or children will assume that the two are somehow linked. If a child feels seriously deprived without a chocolate 'fix' then look at reducing portion sizes rather than banning favourites, perhaps giving a small 'snack size' bar plus some fruit instead of a full-sized one. Create the concept of 'healthy exercise, healthy snack'.

Remember that situations away from home when children are hungry can provide great opportunities for increasing fruit consumption. If there is nothing else available and a child is handed an apple, it will be enjoyed as much as any other snack.

What about children who do not seem interested in getting fit?

Rome wasn't built in a day. Even though a parent may be keen on a household fitness drive, children need time to adjust to new changes to what they do and enjoy. Changing a child's approach to fitness and healthy eating will take months or even years and is a gradual process. Aim for small changes to broaden the things a child enjoys and build on them. A small improvement that becomes a part of life will be far more beneficial than a short burst of hyperactivity that fizzles out in a few weeks.

If new ideas are forced on a child, they will switch off or even become hostile, so involve children in decisions after giving information about the choices on offer.

Invite children to join the family team

Whilst some couch potatoes were simply born with an aversion to getting out of breath, other children lose their early enjoyment of games and sports due to emotional worries or because their poor fitness makes any exercise feel like very hard work.

Either way, all children will be helped by knowing they are part of a team – the family team. Team players know that the rest of the team are there for support and to help out. There is no need to climb mountains alone or unaided – the team can share the load, even if it is made up of a single parent and one child. Family teams might include brothers and sisters, aunts, uncles, cousins and grand-parents, or even an unrelated best friend.

But being part of a team means having responsibilities too. This sometimes means doing what everyone else wants to do, rather than your own first choice. It also means giving support to others when they are struggling. When a parent shares their feelings and troubles with their child, it is a way of showing how much the child is valued and part of the family team. Using the concept of 'the family team' helps with many things such as making a child feel important, helping to practise sports and teaching good family values and habits that can be relied on throughout later life.

Whenever looking to improve lifestyle, start with building on the good things. Work out what the family team is currently doing well at and see what can be added to the list.

Understand worries from a child's point of view

In order to take part in team games or to be seen exercising or keeping fit, people need a degree of self-confidence. No one likes to be laughed at or teased, so it may take courage to join in a game that requires skill or to don a skimpy sports outfit that leaves wobbly bits on display. If a child has already suffered taunts or has felt a failure at games then it is hardly surprising that they may duck out of situations where it may happen again.

Teasing is very common and is not always meant unkindly, but for someone who dreads the situation, even mild leg pulling may appear more like bullying than light-hearted banter. A child in this situation might easily overreact to childish joking, perhaps with tears or an outburst, which may then lead to more teasing. This is the start of a vicious circle, where the child being teased feels tense from the start and becomes more likely to react in a way that makes them a target for more teasing. This then becomes a form of bullying, as others keep teasing just to test out the child's reaction.

From about the age of seven children become increasingly aware of differences between them and their friends, and start to fear personal embarrassment, failing at a task and losing control. Teasing can quickly become a heavy burden, especially since this age group is not old enough to explain to an adult the context in which taunts were said, so that taunts and jibes may be brushed off by teachers or parents, even though they were very hurtful at the time.

All children must learn to cope with disappointment and upset, so the pain of waiting to be chosen (or not) for the rounders team, not being invited to a party or being left out of the school play are all important experiences that teach people to deal with the anxiety–disappointment cycle that happens throughout life. During childhood, parental support can help children to put things in perspective and overcome these obstacles, and deal with the emotions that they bring.

Dealing with bullying

People cope better with problems when they feel good inside, whereas problems seem far worse when feeling low. Whether or not people worry about a problem will depend on whether there is a solution. Even if there is a huge problem on the horizon, it may generate less worry than a tiny problem if the huge one can be sorted, but the tiny one won't go away. People can change how they deal with problems if they feel strong inside, especially if they feel there is more than one solution.

If bullying is the problem, it may seem like a tiny problem when described to others, but it is a tiny one that won't seem to go away, making it feel huge to the victim. Being bullied makes it hard to imagine that there can be a choice in how to respond, but this is a crucial factor in helping a child with low self-confidence. Bullying makes people feel there is no way out, but this is not the case.

Discuss the following factors to help a child understand how things can begin to change.

- Bullies are usually low in self-confidence themselves and pick on their victims as a way of boosting their own fragile image. They only pick on people who they *think* are weaker than themselves: they do not necessarily *know* that their victim is weaker. If bullies find that their victim has hidden strengths then they usually move on to a different victim.

- Bullies like a reaction. They usually do not bother causing trouble if there is no audience, but will go to lengths to play up in front of their friends. If the victim reacts, it usually means that the bully will try again to see if they can get an even bigger reaction.
- Bullies like to make their victim upset as this is a form of victory – it makes the bully feel as though something has been achieved, which is why it boosts their own fragile image. Whilst it can be very difficult not to react and to show hurt feelings – or even hurt flesh – getting no reaction will raise doubts in the bully's mind about whether the victim is a safe 'weak' bet, and they will have failed to impress their friends.
- Whilst it is a good idea to report bullying and get an adult – either a teacher or parent – to come and sort things out, this may be only a temporary cure. Adults can sometimes put a halt to bullying behaviour, but if the bully still thinks that the victim is weaker they will continue to choose moments to taunt when the coast is clear. If adults have become involved, find ways to boost the victim's confidence and inner strength to show the bully that things have changed.
- Inner strength does not have to come from dealing with the current problem. Movies are full of scenarios where the nasty villain gets his comeuppance, but real life is not usually like this. 'Sorting out the bully' would be a great way to boost inner strength, but it is certainly not the only way: inner strength can be boosted despite ongoing bullying. Box 11.3 gives ideas on how to rebuild self-esteem.

Box 11.3 Rebuilding self-esteem

- Have good support from friends and family. This means telling them what is going on, so they know that their help is needed. Bottling things up usually makes problems last longer.
- Be clear about what the problems really are. Sometimes when people are very down, the whole of life feels like it is going wrong. Discussing this in depth together may help a child put things in perspective and see that many things in life are not so bad after all, and the actual problem itself may then seem a bit clearer.
- Show children that parents want to support the child's attempts to improve things, rather than barge in with their own ideas. Many children worry that well-meaning parents will make things worse if they explain what is going on, and so keep quiet about worries and bullying. Give reassurance that parents will only take action with the child's agreement, but they would still like to listen.
- Focus on one really good thing in life and make this factor as special as possible. Examples may be getting a pet; joining a new club out of school, perhaps where no fellow students go; getting involved with a parent's hobby; getting paid for doing something – possibly on a regular basis, such as car washing or helping with chores – and then planning how the money will be spent; being good at a subject. Whilst academic success occasionally means some children will be labelled as swots, they are likely to earn far more money in the long run – and then who will be laughing?
- Gain status from unusual things, and things that people at school can't check up on. For example, if a child were to try canoeing or archery in

the summer, or learn a martial art or self-defence, this could give opportunities for them to boost their profile in a way that can't be double-checked at school. Display certificates, badges or photos as proof of attainment as well as to remind children of their success.

- Explain how sometimes problems do not exactly go away, but people learn to live with them. Looking at problems in the short and longer term can help explain this. For example, if a child was bullied so much that they had to find a new school, there is always the chance that it might begin at the new school too. Finding ways to deflect bullying by building inner strength is a way of learning to live with the problem, rather than running away from it. Working towards lots of 'feel-good' days will give a cushion, so that bullying from the nasty people in life won't be quite such a big deal.

Never ignore signs of real distress in a child

Some situations can trigger depression in a child, just as they can in adults. Some children may cope with all sorts of worries, but then an extra problem will tip them over the edge. For example, a child may struggle with a grandparent's death, or with the separation or divorce of parents. Sometimes the loss of a pet can come as an unexpectedly hard blow. Often people do not realise just how damaging and soul-destroying bullying can be until a child falls apart.

Whilst suicide is very rare in children before puberty, it is not unknown. More commonly, children react by becoming withdrawn and losing interest in sports or games that they used to enjoy, or by starting to use cigarettes, alcohol or even drugs or solvents to block out their misery.

A change in behaviour is a common signal that all is not well, but if a child talks about self-harm or thoughts of wanting to die, this should be taken very seriously. Further help from a family doctor, paediatrician, social worker or possibly the emergency services should be accessed as soon as possible. There is further information about recognising and helping depression in Chapter 15 'An A to Z of conditions that affect eating and weight in younger children'.

Summary points

- Put exercise and activities somewhere on the priority list for both adults and children. Bin the excuses and look for small improvements to daily routines, rather than a short-lived burst of marathon running.
- Make exercise enjoyable or the battle will be lost.
- Raise the profile of activities by involving parents, showing interest and helping out with practising new skills.
- Help children to be organised to take part.
- Explore outside options such as school and clubs for extra activity ideas.
- Use the 'family team' approach to giving children support in getting fitter.
- Look at worries from a child's viewpoint; tackle teasing and bullying if it has become a problem.
- Never ignore real distress in a child.

Section 4

Nutrition and health problems

So far, this book has looked at understanding and putting into practice various principles that govern children's choices and motivation. This understanding allows parents to introduce change in order to boost the whole family's health. Armed with this knowledge, parents can successfully introduce healthier meals and menus. The following chapters take a more detailed look at the building blocks of the diet, healthy foods and how to improve existing family meals and snacks by ensuring that they follow the principles of *The Balance of Good Health*. Illnesses associated with eating tendency or ability to exercise are covered in Chapter 15.

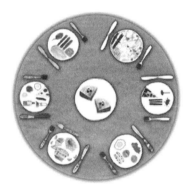

Nutritional nuts and bolts

Facts about fat

Fat has its uses

Despite a national obsession with eating low-fat foods, fat is an essential part of the diet, especially for growing children. It provides energy, insulation to keep the body warm, padding to sit on and is an essential part of many cells in the body, allowing them to function. In addition, some vitamins can only be taken into the body when combined with fat, so it is needed to absorb vitamins A, D, E and K.

Fat is very energy-dense, which means there are lots of calories in a small amount of fat – around twice as many per gram than carbohydrate or protein. Therefore one spoonful of fat will contain the same calories as two spoonfuls of either carbohydrate or protein. This is good for children who have a small appetite because a high-fat diet provides lots of energy without having to eat a lot.

Without fat in the diet, many foods would taste unpleasant. Fat adds a different type of moisture to a food than water, and it is often fat that gives a food its creamy and enjoyable texture. Unfortunately, this is a major reason why so many families struggle with their weight – fat, in combination with many other foods, tastes great, and this can lead to overeating.

Understand why low-fat eating is recommended

After the early years, when a high-fat diet is suitable, children should gradually be encouraged to enjoy lower-fat foods, so that no more than 30% of the calories in the diet come from fat. Most of this fat will be found in dairy products and in some of the protein-containing foods, but some will come from cakes, biscuits and confectionery.

Too much fat is a problem for a variety of reasons:

- Fat is far more energy-dense than protein and carbohydrate, making it easy to overeat because fat triggers the sense of fullness more slowly than both protein and carbohydrate.

Type of food	Calories per gram of food
Protein	4
Fat	9
Carbohydrates	4

- People are not very good at adjusting for a fatty meal whilst eating, but can do so over the course of the day. This is best explained by using an example.

> Pat and Jim both loved spaghetti bolognese. Pat came from a family where everyone was encouraged to clear their plates but Jim's family were happy to leave unwanted food. In both homes spaghetti bolognese was usually prepared with very little oil in the sauce and with extra lean mince. Pat and Jim met up in a restaurant and both ordered spaghetti bolognese for lunch, which tasted similar to home-cooking but contained far more oil and had lots of Parmesan cheese sprinkled on top. Both ate the full plateful, even though this meant eating more calories than they usually did at lunchtime. Neither noticed that the restaurant's meal contained more fat than home cooking. At teatime, Jim found he was far less hungry than usual and was happy to have just a sandwich for tea. He was compensating for the earlier fatty meal. Pat, however, was not used to registering how hungry he was and tucked into his usual tea, so that he ate far more food over the course of the day without realising.

- Too much fat in a diet can push out the healthier items. If children fill up first on fried foods and snacks, there will be less room and less desire for the healthy parts of the diet, such as fruit and vegetables. However, if a meal begins with low-fat foods and fresh produce, with higher-fat items being reserved for the end, the likelihood that the healthy basics are eaten will increase; and because this takes the edge off an appetite, there will be less risk of overeating higher-fat items.

- Although hibernating animals need to fatten themselves up for winter, humans have ready supplies of food all year round and are better off leaving their energy stores in kitchen cupboards rather than tucked around their waists. Carrying too much fat through adulthood has been linked to a whole range of illnesses, as listed in Box 12.1. Diabetes is the likeliest weight-related condition to cause problems. In overweight women, where body mass index (BMI) is between 25 and 30, the chance of diabetes increases by five times. But if BMI is over 35 (which is in the obese range) then the risk of diabetes increases by a staggering 93 times. The picture is very similar for men too.

> **Box 12.1 Illnesses and conditions associated with overweight and obesity**
>
> - Diabetes
> - High blood pressure
> - Stroke
> - Heart attack
> - Heart failure
> - Blood clotting tendency
> - Raised cholesterol level
> - Gallstones
> - Some cancers (of the breast, womb and pancreas)
> - Reduced fertility
> - Osteoarthritis symptoms
> - Breathing problems, in particular whilst asleep
> - Liver problems
> - Depression

Some fats are better than others

If up to 30% of the diet is to be made up of fat, does it matter what sort of fat is eaten? The answer is yes. There are two main types of fat: saturated (usually hard at room temperature) and unsaturated (usually liquid at room temperature). Saturated fat raises cholesterol and increases the risk of heart disease and cancer. Unsaturated fats can lower cholesterol, which can reduce the chance of heart disease. Examples of which fats are found in different foods are given in Table 12.1.

How can families choose lower-fat foods without taking a calculator and textbook to the supermarket?

There are some easy concepts to follow to make lower-fat eating straightforward.

- The list of ingredients can give a rough idea of how much fat a food contains. Ingredients are listed in order of proportion, so the main ones will be listed first. If a fatty ingredient is one of the first two or three items, it is likely to be a higher-fat food. If it is listed at the end of a long list or not at all, the fat content should be very low. Watch out for processed meats though, as they use fatty meat or untrimmed meat rather than lean, so even though the ingredients will list meat, the fat content may still be high.
- Watch out for alternative words used to describe fat on food labels: butter, buttermilk, dripping, lard, milk fat, peanut butter or oil, vegetable oil or fat, any word that ends in 'glycerides'.
- Reserve processed foods such as pies, burgers, sausages and batter-coated meats or fish to once or twice a week only. Avoid the trap of varying the family diet with different processed foods each day, or this will result in a high-fat diet. Choose lean meats (or trim excess fat off fattier cuts), stews and try vegetarian options on occasion.

Table 12.1 Examples of fats found in different foods

Type of fat	Found in
Saturated fats (try to limit)	Visible fat on meat, processed meats, dairy products, lard and some margarines
– Vegetable fat or palm or coconut fat, also known as 'tree lard'!	Pies, pastry, biscuits, cakes and processed foods
– Hydrogenated vegetable oil or fat	Cakes, confectionery, ice-cream, pies, cereal bars, crisps and many other products
– *Trans* fats	These are formed in the manufacture of hydrogenated fat and worsen heart disease risks further
Unsaturated fats (healthier, because they can improve heart disease risks by improving cholesterol)	Usually from plants
– Monounsaturated fat	Olive oil, nuts, seeds, avocados, rape seed oil
– Polyunsaturated fat	Vegetable oils, such as sunflower oil and vegetable oil spreads, oily fish, nuts
– Omega 3 and 6 oils	Omega-3 enriched eggs, oily fish, nuts and seeds, soya beans and vegetable oils

- Choose lower-fat dairy products, such as semi-skimmed or skimmed milk and low-fat yoghurts.

Skimmed milk	0.6g fat per pint
Semi-skimmed milk	9g fat per pint
Full-fat milk	22g fat per pint

- Change cooking methods. Try steaming, boiling, grilling, poaching or micro-waving food, rather than frying or roasting. Deep-frying, in particular, results in a very high fat content because the food becomes soaked in oil.
- Try 'dry-roasting' or a 'dry-fry', which is frying with next to no oil. If some oil is really needed then oil sprays are available that give a fine mist rather than the amount used when pouring from a bottle.
- Make use of the natural oil that is within the food already when frying or roasting. If a recipe calls for onions to be fried first in a little oil and for meat to be added second, try reversing this order: onions can be fried in the oil that comes out of the meat when it is sealed, so that no extra is needed. Alternatively, after using a little oil to begin with, any oil that is not absorbed into the ingredients can be skimmed off later during the cooking process.
- If there are concerns about the family being overweight, reduce all types of fat – saturated and unsaturated – as both are equally full of calories.
- Be sceptical about low-fat claims on packaging: this information is sometimes used to make a product sound healthier than it really is. If in doubt, check out its food label and think about where the item fits on *The Balance of Good Health* plate. Remember that '80% fat free' actually means that 20% of the food *is* fat.
- Use the guide below to judge the fat content that is listed on the food label.

High-fat food	*Low-fat food*
20g fat or more per 100g	3g fat or less per 100g
5g saturates or more per 100g	1g saturates or less per 100g

  If the amount is in between these figures, then it will be a moderately high-fat food.

Make sense of 'sugars'

Everyone thinks of sugar as the sweet granules that are sprinkled on desserts. However, sugar means roughly the same as carbohydrate, so sometimes these terms are interchanged. There are various types of carbohydrates, ranging from simple sugars – ones that taste sweet and dissolve easily – to complex carbo-hydrates such as starch. After they have been eaten, the body breaks all carbo-hydrates down into glucose, which is the main carbohydrate within the body.

Complex carbohydrates are more useful to the body than simple sugars. Glucose on its own is a bit like a lost worker without any tools – the worker might be vaguely useful but isn't organised or well equipped to be really helpful. Unrefined complex carbohydrates, where glucose molecules are stacked together in long chains, are like whole armies of workers all grouped together. Not only are they organised but they come with tools and equipment too – which are fibre, vitamins and minerals. Complex carbohydrates provide essential nutrients in addition to their steady slow release of energy, whereas simple sugars provide only a surge of rapid energy without additional nutrients, which is why they are sometimes called 'empty calories'.

Simple sugars

These occur naturally in food, for example in fruit, some vegetables, cereal grains and milk, and can also be added to food, when they are termed extrinsic or added sugars. As they provide energy but little else, they do not contribute much to a balanced diet.

Limit the amount of added sugars in the overall diet, partly because they are a cause of tooth decay, but also because they are often combined with fat, making them unsuitable for frequent consumption. On food labels they will be listed as 'carbohydrates (of which sugars)'.

Many different words are used on packaging to mean sugar, such as brown sugar, cane sugar, dextrose, fruit sugar, glucose, honey, molasses, syrup and treacle.

A high-sugar food will have at least 10 grams of sugars per 100 grams.

A low-sugar food will have less than 2 grams of sugars per 100 grams.

Complex carbohydrates

These provide a healthy way to fill up without consuming excessive energy, whilst bringing along other essential nutrients too, such as fibre, minerals and vitamins. There are three different types to be aware of: unrefined carbohydrates, refined or processed carbohydrates, and fibre (*see* Table 12.2).

Table 12.2 Types of carbohydrate

Type of carbohydrate	Found in	Essential nutrients they contain
Unrefined carbohydrates	Wholegrain cereals	Fibre
	Wholemeal or granary flour	Protein
	Brown rice	Vitamins B and E
	Potatoes	Minerals: zinc, copper and iron
	Wholewheat pasta	Antioxidants
	Lentils and other pulses	Phytonutrients
	Fruit and vegetables	
Refined or processed carbohydrates	White flour, hence in white bread, pastry, cakes, sugary breakfast cereals	Small amounts of fibre
		Small amounts of vitamins and minerals
Fibre (also known as non-starch polysaccharides or NSP)	Fruit and vegetables, especially coconut	Roughage that helps the gut to work smoothly
	Wholegrain cereals and flour	Helps to keep moisture within the gut, which keeps motions soft
	Bran-enriched cereals	
	Beans and other pulses	
	Nuts	

Unrefined carbohydrates

These tend to be eaten in much the same form that they were harvested, so that very few of their nutrients have been lost in processing by the time they are eaten. They are the healthiest form of carbohydrate because in addition to plenty of fibre, they contain protein, vitamins B and E, minerals (such as zinc, copper and iron), antioxidants and phytonutrients. These last two are substances that help body cells to resist damage from pollutants and toxins. Unrefined carbohydrates have a low glycaemic index, or GI, which means they are broken down and absorbed slowly in the gut, so they are able to keep hunger at bay for longer than refined carbohydrates or simple sugars.

Refined or processed carbohydrates

Examples include white flour and bread, cakes and low-fibre breakfast cereals. Not only do these carbohydrates lose many nutrients in the refining process, they are often combined with added sugar and fat, resulting in tempting and tasty foods that upset the balance of a good diet. The body is able to absorb them quickly into the bloodstream (which is shown by a high glycaemic index), giving a rapid surge in blood sugar but then an equally rapid fall again, so that hunger may not be staved off for long. Where possible they should be swapped for wholegrain options.

Fibre

The body is unable to digest dietary fibre so, instead of providing energy, it helps the gut to work by increasing bulk in the bowel and by stimulating the gut walls. Many foods contain fibre, especially wholegrain foods, but some contain particularly high amounts, such as fresh or desiccated coconut, high-bran breakfast cereals, baked beans, red kidney beans and other pulses. Choosing plenty of wholegrain foods and fresh produce should ensure that the diet contains plenty of fibre without necessarily needing to eat high-bran breakfast cereals. However, some people have trouble with constipation despite eating a range of healthy foods, in which case a high-fibre breakfast cereal can be a simple way to overcome the problem. It can also improve tummy symptoms in the short term whilst experimenting to see which other foods will achieve the same improvement, as this can take a little while. Because extra fibre can cure abdominal pains, it could be described as a 'healing' food, with a high-fibre breakfast cereal acting as a dose of medicine!

How much fibre should children eat?

Whilst adults are advised to eat around 18 grams of fibre each day, this amount varies between individuals. Some people eat far more and others eat less; the 'right' amount depends on the ease with which a person's digestive system works. If this is causing problems then more fibre is usually a good idea.

For children, the 'right' amount varies in much the same way. Some children need more fibre than others, but many children hardly eat any fibre at all. If a child strains when visiting the loo or suffers colicky tummy pains then the fibre in their diet is inadequate. There is a surprising number of people who have always suffered discomfort from their bowels, but because it has been a lifelong problem they believe that this pattern is normal. Just because family tendencies suggest a

Table 12.3 Dietary fibre guide for common foods

Food		Average portion size	Grams of fibre per portion
Breakfast cereals:	High-bran cereal	30 g (or 1 small	8.1
	Bran Flakes	bowl)	4.5
	Weetabix	2	4.0
	Malted wheat/Shreddies		3.6
	Corn Flakes*		0.9
	Rice Crispies*		0.45
Bread:	Wholemeal	2 slices (47 g)	3.5
	Brown		2.8
	White		1.8
Vegetables:	Peas	2 heaped	3.2
	Broccoli	tablespoons	1.8
	Carrots		1.5
	Runner beans		2.2
Fruit:	Satsumas	2 (100 g)	1.3
	Apple	1 (150 g)	3.0
	Banana	1 (120 g)	3.7
	Peach	1 (120 g)	1.8
Potatoes:	Jacket	180 g	4.9
	Boiled	180 g	2.2
Rice:	Brown	180 g	1.4
	White*	180 g	0.2
Beans and pulses:	Baked beans	200 g (half can)	7.4
	Red kidney beans	3 tablespoons	7.7
	Red lentils	3 tablespoons	2.2

* Lower-fibre foods for comparison.

weekly motion is the norm does not mean that this norm is healthy, and small changes to the general diet can make a big difference to bowel habits.

Children will benefit from developing a taste for, or at least tolerance of, higher-fibre foods, so that if their systems need additional fibre they will be happy to choose suitable foods to provide this. As children grow older they should aim to eat roughly the same amount of fibre as adults, which is around 18 grams a day. Young children do not need as much because their appetites are proportionately smaller and high-fibre foods tend to be bulky. Hence a very high-fibre diet might leave a child feeling full before enough food has been eaten. If a young child needs more fibre because of constipation, then eating higher-fat foods (such as full-fat milk and extra butter on bread) alongside the extra fibre can help to overcome a small appetite.

Table 12.3 lists good sources of dietary fibre plus some lower-fibre foods (marked with an asterisk) for comparison.

Protein puzzles

There is a lot of confusion about protein because humans need a variety of different proteins for good health. The secret, as ever, lies in eating a varied diet so that all individual protein building blocks (otherwise known as amino acids) are consumed. There is nothing particularly special about protein that comes from meat – most proteins ultimately come from plants. All the protein in a nice juicy steak was obtained from grass in the cow's diet. Vegetarians should have no problem in finding all the proteins that are needed to keep them healthy, as long as they eat a varied diet.

If excessive protein is eaten it does not produce extra muscle. The amount of muscle bulk created depends on how much muscles are used and exercised, plus the effects of hormones (such as insulin and growth hormone), rather than how much protein is eaten. Any extra protein that is not used up in building muscles, making hormones or cell repair will be burned as fuel or laid down as fat. Humans do not store extra protein in the way that excess fat is stored.

Because children are growing they need a higher proportion of protein than adults, and should aim to eat about 1 gram per kilogram of body weight each day. This means that a child weighing 30 kg should eat about 30 grams of protein from several different sources each day. Adults will get by on around 0.75 grams per kilogram of body weight.

Table 12.4 Percentage of energy from protein-containing foods

Protein-containing foods	% of energy from protein
Tuna, tinned in brine	95
Baked cod	89
Roast chicken	75
Boiled ham slices	53
Broccoli	52
Cheddar cheese, reduced fat	48
Cauliflower, raw	42
Boiled egg	35
Peas	35
Red lentils, boiled	30
Semi-skimmed milk	29
Baked beans	25
Cheddar cheese, full fat	25
Yoghurt	20
Peanuts	17
Wholemeal bread	17
Pasta	15
White bread	14
Custard (carton)	11
Boiled potato	10
Carrots, boiled	10
Cornflakes	9
Boiled rice	8
Chocolate	6
Banana	5
Apple, eating	3

How can families be sure they are eating sufficient protein?

Proteins are in all sorts of foods, as shown in Table 12.4, so if the family diet is reasonably varied then it will provide different sources of protein. There are 20 different protein building blocks or amino acids, which can be grouped in a huge variety of ways to make different proteins. Humans can manufacture some but not all of these building blocks, which means that the ones that can't be made are essential in the diet. This is why a varied diet is so important – some protein foods are good for some of the building blocks, but not others. A varied diet will ensure they are all eaten one way or the other.

Take a look at the list of foods in Table 12.4 to see how much of their energy is in the form of protein.

As the list shows, protein provides a proportion of energy in foods that may not usually be thought of as a source of protein, such as pasta. If a person eats large amounts of pasta then this will provide a fair amount of protein. Some vegetables are surprisingly high in protein, such as broccoli and peas. Be aware that some good sources of protein also contain high fat levels too, such as full-fat cheese, whereas choosing a reduced-fat cheese means more protein per mouthful.

Traditional food combinations have developed in many communities which help to balance essential amino acids, often by combining plant with animal proteins, especially milk, which contains almost all of the building blocks that humans require. These combinations mean that any of the essential building blocks not found in one ingredient will appear in the other. Some examples are beans on toast, macaroni cheese, rice pudding, breakfast cereal with milk, lentil curry with rice, tortillas and beans.

Five-a-day fruit and vegetables

Looking at *The Balance of Good Health*, a third of the daily diet should be in the form of fruit and vegetables, but that doesn't mean the nation must endure a lifetime of rabbit food! On the contrary, fruit and vegetables are highly versatile,

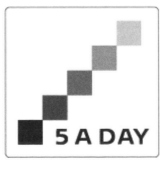

5 A DAY

Just Eat More
(fruit & veg)

Figure 12.1 '5 A Day'. Reproduced by kind permission of the Department of Health.

with many cheap varieties that can be easily incorporated into family meals and snacks.

Some food manufacturers and supermarkets are now labelling packaging with the 'five-a-day' logo (*see* Figure 12.1), which helps to show how many portions of fruit and vegetables a typical serving of the food contains. If the logo appears on a packet it confirms that at least one portion of fruit or vegetable is within. If more than one of the little boxes are coloured in then it shows that one serving counts as two (or more) portions.

Why are fruit and vegetables so great?

Firstly, they are a very natural thing to eat. Humans evolved as 'grazing omnivores', which means our ancestors would eat anything edible that was available, whether meat or plant food. Unlike lions, for example, that gorge every few days on a meat kill, humans learned to grab any opportunity to eat anything vaguely palatable, such as berries, fruit, nuts and grains, in addition to meat. By evolving to make use of nutrients from varied sources, humans became very adept at survival. Even though humans no longer graze particularly, instead following community habits by eating at set meal times, most are still usually omnivores. The essentials of the human diet are easiest to obtain by eating meat, cereal foods, and fruit and vegetables, rather than pinning all hopes on only one food group as lions do.

Secondly, fruit and vegetables are ideal for filling up healthily without any worry about eating too much. Looking again at *The Balance of Good Health*, if the fruit and vegetable segment is missed out, then other foods are eaten in greater amounts, which usually means eating more 'junk' foods so that calorie intake goes up. Putting fruit and veg back in means pushing some of the less healthy foods 'off the plate' (*see* Figure 12.2).

Thirdly, as already mentioned, fruit and vegetables are an excellent source of vitamins, minerals, fibre, antioxidants and phytonutrients. More fruit and veg means less heart disease and cancer.

What about portion sizes for children?

Whilst scientists have worked out formulas for ideal portion sizes for adults, looking at *The Balance of Good Health* there is no fixed amount that is correct – what matters is the proportion of mouthfuls that come from fruit and vegetables compared to other types of food, which should be about one-third. However, it can help to have a rough idea of an average adult's portion sizes and some guidance about amounts for children. More importantly, if children are encouraged to enjoy fruit and vegetables, then this enjoyment will lead them to choose as much as they want – which might be far more than the minimum five-a-day recommended amounts. Forcing fruit or vegetables is pointless and may put children off for good.

Adult portions of fruit or vegetables are roughly 80 grams (or 3 ounces), which works out as about three tablespoons of chopped vegetables, a cereal bowlful of salad or one whole fruit such as an apple, orange or banana. For children, the amount is reduced according to appetite: if a child eats roughly half the volume of

(a)

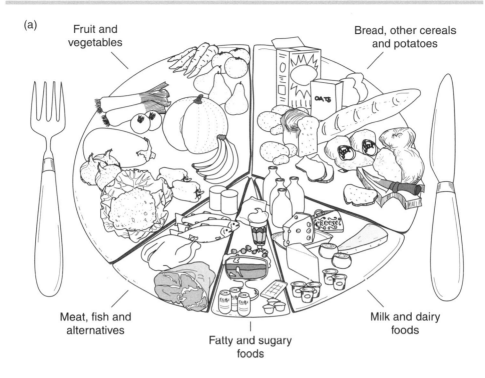

Fruit and
vegetables

Bread, other cereals
and potatoes

Meat, fish and
alternatives

Fatty and sugary
foods

Milk and dairy
foods

(b)

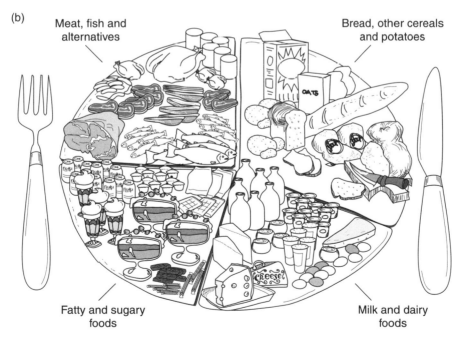

Meat, fish and
alternatives

Bread, other cereals
and potatoes

Fatty and sugary
foods

Milk and dairy
foods

Figure 12.2 *The Balance of Good Health* (a) with fruit and vegetables and (b) without.

Table 12.5 Rough guide to portion sizes

Adult and child over age 11	1 portion = 3 tablespoons
Child aged 5 to 11	1 portion = 3 dessertspoons
Child aged 2 to 5	1 portion = 3 teaspoons
Child aged up to 2	1 portion = any little mouthfuls to encourage familiarity and enjoyment of the food

food as an adult then the fruit and vegetable portions will also be roughly half (*see* Table 12.5).

Another way to work this is by thinking of a 'portion' as the amount that fits in the palm of the hand. Big hands: big portions. Small hands: small portions!

How do other items fit into the five-a-day plan?

- Fruit and vegetables count towards each day's quota regardless of whether they are raw, frozen, cooked, chilled, canned or dried. Vegetables within a stew or takeaway count too.
- Even fruit that is past its best can be blended into a smoothie to count as a portion.
- Whilst it is best to have five portions of different produce, this is not essential and some servings will count as two portions, such as cauliflower cheese served as a main course.
- Some items, however, only count as one portion, however much is served. An example is fruit juice, which counts as one portion even if several glasses are drunk, because part of the fruit is left behind during the juicing process, leaving it with very little fibre.
- Pulse vegetables and beans such as chickpeas, lentils and kidney beans also only count as one portion per day, regardless of amount, because whilst good for fibre, they are not so good for vitamins and minerals.
- Portion sizes of dried fruit such as raisins, apricots and dates are smaller than fresh portions because even though they lose moisture during the drying process, the other sugars and nutrients become more concentrated. One spoonful rather than three counts as a portion, but only one portion counts each day.
- Potatoes do not count as fruit or veg at all because they are counted in the carbohydrate group along with rice, pasta and bread.

Tips for making fruit a success

It is very disappointing to choose a shiny green apple only to find it hard and bitter. A child's early experiences of unripe or impossible-to-peel fruit could make fruit in general seem like hard work. Teach children how to choose the right item from a selection and take a little trouble to make it appear appealing:

- Fruit needs to be ripe in order for it to taste good. Peaches, nectarines, plums, strawberries, grapefruit and melon give off a sweet smell when they are ready for eating, whereas some fruits tend to give off their smell only when they are a bit over-ripe, such as kiwis, bananas and pineapple. All of these fruits, plus pears, can also be checked for ripeness by pressing very gently on the surface. If it yields slightly then the fruit will be ripe, but if hard then it should be left for a few more days to ripen before trying again.

- Fruit is more likely to ripen well in the right season. For example, imported strawberries at Christmas are often a disappointment whereas they are far more enjoyable in the summer.
- Apples can be tricky to tell if ripe. If in doubt then leave apples longer at room temperature and they will ripen a little more. Apples that are getting old tend to lose their shine and may become slightly shrivelled, but the flesh inside is often even sweeter at this stage.
- It can be hard to tell if oranges will be sweet or rather tangy and bitter. In general, the smaller fruit such as clementines, satsumas and mandarin oranges are easier for children to peel and more reliably sweet. Larger oranges with thicker skins can be delicious, but children might require help to peel them. Young children will not help themselves to fruit from the fruit bowl if fiddly peeling is required.
- Wobbly front teeth can make eating an apple or pear a nightmare. Chop them up or offer an alternative during this phase of childhood.
- Many children will react violently to unsightly blemishes, bruises or the presence of grubs in fruit. Teach them to tolerate small blemishes and to cut out bruised areas of fruit, rather than wasting it all. If this approach is unsuccessful then cut up imperfect fruit to make a fruit salad, adding several types, which can include dried or tinned fruit, for interest and texture.
- Fruit that has been chopped up and put on the table is far more likely to be eaten than if left whole in the fruit bowl.

Tips for vegetables

- Rather than only serving vegetables on their own, they can be thrown in with other foods such as cook-in sauces.
- Vegetables taste great when very lightly cooked so they are still crunchy, such as in a stir-fry. Adding herbs, garlic, Worcestershire sauce or some lemon juice can give them extra flavour.
- Do not underestimate raw vegetables. Boost a plain salad with sliced or grated carrot, small broccoli florets, sugar snap peas, a tin of sweet corn or even frozen peas that have been allowed to thaw. Raw mushroom has an unusual texture and delicate flavour, as do baby corn cobs, which can be eaten raw, cooked or straight from the tin.
- Although potatoes do not count as vegetables because they fit into the starch category, swede or carrot added to mash will count.
- Leftover vegetables can be dry-fried the next day with a few fresh ingredients or a bit of bacon or chicken for an easy meal.
- If a recipe calls for onion, then leek can be used instead or in addition to increase vegetable portions.

Further ideas on using fruit and vegetables to improve the balance of family meals are given in Chapter 13.

Dairy products

There should be around three portions of dairy products and milk in the daily diet for both adults and children, where one portion is about one-third of a pint (200 ml). There may be confusion about dairy products because they are often a source of fat as well as calcium and protein, and so some adults may have tried to reduce intake to help their own weight. Young children need fat because it is an important source of energy for 'small eaters', and so full-fat dairy products are fine. As children grow and eat larger volumes of food, moving onto lower-fat dairy products is better unless a child is doing high levels of sport, requiring extra energy.

Full-fat milk and dairy products – use up to age five then move to lower-fat options

Semi-skimmed milk – can be introduced over the age of two if the child has a good appetite

Skimmed milk – reserve until over the age of five

Encouragingly, low-fat dairy products have just as much calcium as full-fat and may have higher amounts of protein per gram.

Calcium is needed for growing bones and teeth. Milk and dairy products are an excellent source of protein, providing almost all of the essential building blocks that are needed in the diet. Children should aim for the equivalent of a pint of milk per day, which can be made up of milk to drink, on cereals or mixed in other foods, plus cheese, yoghurt and fromage frais.

Occasionally, a child may appear to be sensitive to dairy products, which is usually shown by marked eczema or severe asthma. If there is a suspicion that eczema or asthma is worsened by a child's diet, this should be discussed further with a family doctor, paediatrician or dietician, to ensure that a diet without dairy products will still provide all the essentials that a growing child needs. There are more details about dairy-free eating in Chapter 14 'Vegetarian and vegan eating'.

Vitamins and minerals

What are vitamins?

Vitamins are essential nutrients that the body needs in small amounts to work properly. There are two types of vitamins: fat-soluble and water-soluble. Fat-soluble vitamins can be stored in the body in the liver and in fat, which means that, whilst they are needed in the diet, they are not essential every day. However, water-soluble vitamins cannot be stored, which means that they do need to be eaten daily.

All vitamins should be obtainable through a varied and balanced diet so that vitamin supplements are not a necessity. However, for children under five who may eat only small amounts or from a limited range of foods, it is recommended to give additional vitamin supplements. Further information about obtaining

Table 12.6 Fat-soluble vitamins

Vitamin	Needed for	Found in
Vitamin A	Night vision, growth, immune system, antioxidant. Deficiency leads to night blindness.	Liver, eggs, oily fish, dairy products and fortified margarine. The body can also manufacture it from beta-carotene, found in yellow and green leafy vegetables such as spinach, carrots and red peppers, and yellow fruit such as mango, melon and apricots.
Vitamin D	Regulates calcium levels in the body and helps bone strength. Deficiency leads to rickets.	Most vitamin D is made in the skin using sunlight, but some is needed in the diet. Found in oily fish, liver, eggs, fortified foods such as margarine, breakfast cereals, bread and powdered milk.
Vitamin E	It is an antioxidant, which helps to protect cell membranes. Deficiency is rare.	Vegetable oils, leafy green vegetables, fruit, nuts and wholegrain cereals.
Vitamin K	Used in blood clotting and for bone strength. Deficiency rare, apart from bleeding disorder of newborn babies.	Leafy green vegetables, vegetable oils and cereals. Small amounts in meat and dairy foods. It is also produced by bacteria in the intestines. Vitamin K is usually given to newborn babies.

vitamin supplements is given in Chapter 4. Giving a vitamin supplement does not take away the need for a balanced diet and will not make a diet of excess sugar or fat any healthier!

Many staple foods are fortified with additional vitamins and minerals, making it easier to obtain the right amounts. Examples include many types of breakfast cereals, certain types of flour, vegetable spreads and margarine.

Fat-soluble vitamins

Fat-soluble vitamins are found mainly in fatty foods such as animal fats (including butter and lard), vegetable oils, dairy foods, liver and oily fish (*see* Table 12.6). They are not destroyed by heating or cooking.

Because the body is able to store these types of vitamins it is also able to take on board too much, so that in excess they can actually lead to harm. It is therefore not advised to overdose on supplements. It is very unlikely that a person could overdose on these vitamins just by eating a balanced diet.

Water-soluble vitamins

The body is not able to store water-soluble vitamins so they need to be eaten frequently. If too much is eaten the body gets rid of any extra vitamins in the urine, so they are not harmful.

Water-soluble vitamins are found in fruit, vegetables and grains (*see* Table 12.7), but they can be destroyed by heat or by being exposed to the air. They can

Table 12.7 Water-soluble vitamins

Vitamin	Needed for	Found in
Vitamin B_6	Energy release from protein and carbohydrate and for blood manufacture. Deficiency can lead to anaemia.	Meat, fish, bread, eggs, wholegrain cereals, vegetables, soya beans, peanuts, milk, potatoes and some fortified breakfast cereals.
Vitamin B_{12}	Works with folic acid to make healthy red blood cells and for the nervous system. Deficiency leads to pernicious anaemia.	Only found in animal foods, especially meat, fish and dairy products, but not plant foods.
Vitamin C	Needed for iron absorption and for keeping cells healthy. Deficiency leads to scurvy.	Most fruit and vegetables, especially broccoli, Brussels sprouts, peppers, kiwi and oranges.
Folic acid	Healthy red blood cell formation. Essential during development of the spine in the fetus.	Broccoli, Brussels sprouts, chickpeas, peas, yeast, oranges and bananas plus many fortified cereals. 400 mcg supplements advised in early pregnancy.
Niacin	Energy release from food, and for healthy cells.	Meat, flour, eggs and milk.
Riboflavin	Energy release and metabolism.	Milk, meat, eggs, fortified breakfast cereal and rice.
Thiamin	Nerve function and for energy release. Deficiency leads to disease of the nervous system.	Dairy products, meat, fortified cereals and flour, fresh and dried fruit.

also be lost in the water used for cooking. Therefore the best way to serve these foods is raw, steamed or grilled rather than boiled.

What are minerals?

Minerals are essential nutrients that are required in small amounts in the form they are found in food. They are found in varying amounts in a variety of foods such as meat, cereals (including cereal products such as bread), fish, milk and dairy foods, vegetables, fruit (especially dried fruit) and nuts. A varied and balanced diet will ensure that adequate minerals are taken in.

Minerals are used for building strong bones and teeth, controlling body fluids inside and outside cells, and turning food into energy.

A brief guide to essential minerals is given in Table 12.8.

What are trace elements?

Trace elements are also essential nutrients that the body needs, but in much smaller amounts than vitamins and minerals. They are found in small amounts in a variety of foods such as meat, fish, cereals, milk and dairy foods, vegetables and nuts. A few examples are given in Table 12.9.

Table 12.8 Essential minerals

Essential mineral	Used for
Calcium	Strong bones and teeth and for blood clotting.
Iron	Fundamental part of haemoglobin, carrying oxygen in the blood.
Magnesium	Needed for bones and for cell walls.
Phosphorus	Required in bones.
Potassium	Essential for fluid control and nerve conduction.
Sodium	Essential for fluid control and blood volume.
Sulphur	Required for removing waste via the liver and for making protein.

Table 12.9 Trace elements

Trace element	Details
Copper	Important for early infant growth and development.
Fluoride	Needed for the enamel on teeth and will reduce tooth decay. Found in toothpaste and in the water supply in some areas.
Iodine	Used by the thyroid gland. Found in seafood and milk.
Zinc	Helps cell growth and wound healing.

Food additives and E-numbers

The whole issue of food additives, particularly in foods targeted at children, is complex and confusing. This short section aims to explore some of the arguments (on both sides), find some reassurance for those parents who find additives hard to avoid and provide sources of further information for families who wish to find out more.

What are E-numbers?

E-numbers form the European classification that is used to identify all additives that go into foods. All of these additives undergo testing to ensure they are safe for people to eat (but not everyone agrees with the conclusions of some of these safety committees).

Table 12.10 lists the different types of additives commonly used and what they are used for.

Some E-numbers are natural ingredients such as salt, but others are synthetic and have been created to improve the convenience factor and attractiveness of food. Studies have shown that the more a food is advertised, the more likely it will contain high amounts of additives. Also, foods with a high fat and/or sugar

Table 12.10 Food additives

Additive category	Reason for use
Preservatives	Stop micro-organisms from making food go off.
Antioxidants	Prevent oils and fats from going rancid.
Gelling agents and stabilisers	Create the desired texture and consistency of foods such as ice cream, yoghurt and salad dressings.
Emulsifiers	Help fats and oils to combine with water within food such as chocolate.
Flavouring agents	Help create the right flavour, especially in soft drinks, soups and sauces.
Colours	Recreate colours in processed foods that have been altered or lost during processing.
Intense sweeteners	Provide sweetness with fewer or no calories.
Acids	Help create the sharpness of certain flavours.

content are far more likely to contain lots of additives than healthier low-fat, low-salt and low-sugar foods.

E-numbers *per se* are not poisonous or toxic, but there are concerns about their overuse in food manufacturing because they make unhealthy food more attractive and they are often used to cover up nutritionally poor basic ingredients by adding in artificial flavouring that has not come from the food itself. An example is chicken nuggets made from mechanically reclaimed meat. Without flavourings and additives these nuggets would be inedible.

It is of even more concern that targeting these types of foods specifically at children helps them to develop a 'taste' for nutritionally poor foods from early on.

There is frequently poor labelling of foods so that the amount of additives is not clear. Some manufacturers list E-numbers themselves and others list the full name of the ingredient so that it may not be clear that the item listed is a food additive.

Table 12.11 lists some of the advantages and disadvantages of food additives.

Table 12.11 Advantages and disadvantages of food additives

Advantages of additives	Disadvantages of additives
Must pass a safety assessment, carried out in many different countries, which is usually reviewed if new information comes to light.	Powerful food organisations are sometimes able to sway the interpretation of safety studies to allow additives to be approved.
They prolong the shelf-life and food quality and reduce the risks of food poisoning.	They are used to make poor ingredients appear better by improving colour and flavour artificially.
They make many foods more appealing.	They can make poor foods more appealing.
They can reduce the cost and improve accessibility of foods by prolonging shelf-life.	They make nutritionally poorer foods more accessible and cheaper due to longer shelf-life.

Controversial additives

It was not until the 1970s that scientists began to suspect a link between food additives and some health and behaviour problems. There has been extensive research into some areas, but because of the nature of symptoms, which are often non-specific and can be caused by several different factors, it can be very hard to prove that a food additive is the true cause of a problem. For example, despite anecdotal evidence (where one or two individuals feel sure that they can see a clear link) that an additive causes childhood behaviour problems, the link becomes much less clear when a large trial is organised, because all sorts of things influence child behaviour. This sort of trial does not confirm or refute the link – it is just not possible to be sure.

Tartrazine: E102

Tartrazine is a synthetic yellow food colouring used in many soft drinks, cakes, sweets, cereals, snacks and desserts. Despite reviews and government-funded surveys which have raised doubts, it is still approved and used widely in the UK, although it has been banned in Norway and Austria. It has been linked with rashes, asthma and hyperactivity in children, although the evidence for this is not clear-cut, as explained above. Food industry pressure has kept it on the approved list because it is such a useful additive.

Other additives that have been linked to hyperactivity in children are E110 (sunset yellow), E124 (ponceau 4 R), E122 (carmosine) and E211 (sodium benzoate). It has been suggested by respected sources that some 25% of temper tantrums in toddlers could be attributed to food additives, but once again it is hard to prove that one thing in particular is the cause when so many things can affect a child's behaviour.

For parents who are in doubt, the most sensible thing is to try reducing or excluding as many additives as possible for a trial period of around two weeks (*see* Table 12.12). For this to be successful, the child should be monitored for a few weeks *before* the exclusion trial so that a baseline of behaviour can be noted down. Then see if there is a noticeable change in, for example, frequency of outbursts, sleep pattern or ability to concentrate on a task. If parents are able to see a

Table 12.12 Common problem foods and good alternatives

Problem foods	Good alternatives
Fizzy drinks, squash	Water, dilute fruit juice, milk, tea without sugar
Fish fingers	Cod or salmon fillet, baked or steamed
Chicken nuggets	Stir-fried chicken strips or home-made nuggets of chicken breast dipped in beaten egg and breadcrumbs
Burgers	Home-made burgers from lean ground beef or a thin strip of frying steak
Flavoured crisps	Ready salted crisps
Yellow custard	Colour-free varieties or choose plain yoghurt with a little added sugar instead

difference then it doesn't matter what the scientists say – stick to the improved foods and keep the problem foods off the menu as much as possible.

Table 12.12 lists some common problem foods, but there are many more processed foods that are brimming with additives – it is necessary to read food labels and develop a basic knowledge of additive-free items if the trial is to be a success. Wherever possible, prepare foods from scratch because then it will be clear what the food is made from.

Further information is available from The Food Commission and through the Hyperactive Children's Support Group (*see* Appendix 2 for further details).

Aspartame: E951

Aspartame is also known as NutraSweet and Canderel and is about 200 times sweeter than sugar. It is used in a huge variety of 'diet' or 'light' products, including fizzy drinks, to create calorie-free sweetness. It has been controversial because there have been claims that it can cause cancer, hair loss, depression, behaviour problems and epilepsy. However, it has been extensively studied by safety committees in America, Europe and other countries and has not been found to be harmful in normal daily intakes.

The lobbyists who support aspartame use the claim that it reduces sugar intake and so should help to reduce diabetes, obesity and tooth decay. In practice, these benefits are as hard to prove as the claims that it causes harm. Whilst, at first glance, a calorie-free sweetener should achieve these aims, in practice, both sugar and sugar-replacement foods encourage the development of a 'sweet tooth' and 'sweet teeth' tend to eat anything sweet on offer without always questioning the calories within. It is always preferable to help children to enjoy varied things, including unsweetened drinks and water, rather than going along with the misconception that sweetness is the key to happiness.

Summary points

- Fat should make up around 30% of the diet for children over the age of five. Up to five years a higher proportion may be suitable for children with a poor appetite.
- Choose healthy fats such as mono- and polyunsaturated fats and omega 3 and 6 oils. Reduce the amount of hard, saturated fats, trans fats and hydrogenated oils and fats.
- Choose plenty of complex, starchy, unrefined carbohydrates to maximise vitamins, minerals and fibre. Reduce sweet, simple sugars as these are 'empty' calories.
- Eat a wide variety of protein-containing foods in order to get the full range of essential protein building blocks, or amino acids. Protein is found in many foods, not just meat.
- Fruit and vegetables should make up a third of the daily diet. Find ways to fit these into existing meals to increase the amount the family eats.
- Low-fat dairy products are just as good a source of calcium as full-fat ones.
- Be confident that some additives are beneficial, whilst taking steps to cut out poor foods that require colourants or flavourings to make them palatable.

Chapter 13

The Food Frequency Framework

Find out which family meals are fine for every day and which should either be put on the 'specials' list or modified in order to become healthy daily meals. Work out which snacks fit the occasion and use portion size to keep fattening favourites from becoming a problem.

Ordinary meals are okay

As studies have shown, children's expectations at mealtimes are not that high and they are happy to eat healthy foods if they are familiar. They are expecting a meal, not an all-singing, all-dancing food extravaganza. Kids have faith in their parents to provide reasonable food. Hence parents can create a basic framework of family meals that are nutritious and healthy, whilst reserving the rich and more elaborate foods for weekends or special occasions when it will be more appropriate to get extra pleasure from food.

By helping children to tune in to their natural appetite and tolerate a wide variety of foods it will be easier to make ordinary meals healthier, and this will result in children who are happy with healthy foods when they are served and who choose healthy things even if there are richer foods on offer.

Referring back to *The Balance of Good Health* in Chapter 1, two-thirds of the plate should be made up of fruit and vegetables and starchy foods. Fruit and vegetables can be fresh, cooked, tinned or frozen, and starchy things include cereals, breads (including chapatti and pitta bread), pasta, rice, potatoes, noodles and couscous. The remaining third of a basic diet should be made up of dairy products and protein-containing foods, plus a small amount of richer, fatty foods or treat-type things. Some examples of protein-containing foods are meat, fish (tinned as well as fresh), eggs and pulses. Pulses include things like baked beans, kidney beans and lentils, which form important sources of protein for vegetarians. The more these ordinary meals fit in with *The Balance of Good Health*, the more freedom this gives to eat richly on special occasions. If the basic diet contains plenty of goodness then the odd 'junk food day' won't matter.

Puddings, if provided, are part of the meal, not an optional extra for good behaviour, and can be a way of adding in extra fruit, dairy or starchy ingredients. Puddings do not have to be overly sweet or sticky, especially on ordinary days, and should fit in with *The Balance of Good Health* just as much as the main course.

What is the Food Frequency Framework?

How often is it okay to eat cheesecake? Or waffles soaked in maple syrup? Or cookie-dough ice-cream? What about roast beef with Yorkshire puddings and all the trimmings? How about chicken nuggets or burgers? All of these common foods have their place, but many foods are not suitable for daily consumption, however tasty they may be.

The Food Frequency Framework shows how to decide which foods are suitable for everyday meals, which are better kept for once-weekly enjoyment and which are best reserved for special occasions or times when food is the centre of the feast. It also gives ideas on how to make family favourites healthy enough to be served frequently, if they are currently falling into one of the richer categories. Portion size is covered later in the chapter.

Table 13.1 shows what factors lead a food to be in one category or another.

Table 13.1 The factors that lead a food to be in one category or another

Celebration foods or rare treats	Once-weekly or weekend foods	Daily basics
Nutrition is simply not an issue.	There is a compromise between convenience or flavour and the food's nutritional value.	Nutrition is important and these foods all have some benefit within the diet.
May contain a high proportion of 'bad' fats such as saturated or trans fats.*	May be moderately high in fat or have some 'bad' fats.	Either low- or no-fat foods, or high in omega 3 and 6 oils or other unsaturated fats.
Expensive or requires lots of time and effort to prepare. May be elaborately packaged.	Moderately expensive or fiddly to prepare. Alternately, its higher cost is offset by its convenience.	Plain ingredients that may be cheap†, with little in the way of fancy packaging.
Requires advanced cooking skills or is available ready prepared, but at a price.	Highly convenient foods that simply require heating up.	Requires basic cooking skills to prepare ingredients.
May be highly decorated or ornate.	May have some decorative features that make the food attractive.	Plain foods with little decoration.
May be high in additives and E-numbers.	May contain some additives and E-numbers.	Will have very few additives.
Usually highly processed ingredients, resulting in very low vitamin, mineral and fibre content.	May contain added vitamins and a little fibre, but their benefit offset by high sugar or fat content.	Unrefined foods containing complex carbohydrates and good levels of vitamins, minerals and fibre.
Do not fit into *The Balance of Good Health* – so keep for special occasions when it doesn't matter.	Can be modified or improved to fit *The Balance of Good Health*.	Fit very well into *The Balance of Good Health*.

* See Chapter 12 for details about different types of fat.
† Many basic ingredients are very cheap, although good sources of protein such as meat and fish tend to be more expensive, as do exotic fruits and vegetables.

From Table 13.1, it can be seen that there are roughly five questions to ask about a food when deciding what it is suitable for:

- Is it cheap or expensive?
- Does it require elaborate preparation or is it easy to prepare?
- Is it a high fat and/or sugar food?
- Does it contain vitamins, minerals or some fibre?
- What about its enjoyment value?

The answers should help to place foods in the right category and so guide how often they can be served. Alternatively, a favourite food can be modified in order to become more nutritious, so that it becomes suitable for eating more frequently. The third way to improve the family diet is by reducing portion sizes of rich foods and padding out meals with more nutritious ingredients, so that they fit better with *The Balance of Good Health*.

Examples of how to fit savoury foods into the three frequency categories

Table 13.2 gives examples of how to fit savoury foods into the three frequency categories.

The list looks at some examples of common family foods, assessing a combination of flavour, convenience of preparation, nutrition, fat content and cost. It is by no means an absolute guide and many families may disagree with how some foods are positioned in the table. This doesn't matter because it is more important for families to decide on the position of their own family favourites, using the guide for ideas. But once decided then this should guide how often the family eats those foods. Families should make some changes if they realise that most of their meals fit into the 'weekend foods' category. It is asking for trouble if a different 'weekend food' appears every day of the week apart from Sundays when a celebration food is chosen!

If too many weekend foods are currently on the week's list, they do not automatically have to be abandoned. The next section looks at ways of improving existing meals.

Tips for turning 'weekend foods' into 'daily basics'

There are three approaches that can help to introduce more nutrition and result in fewer undesirable ingredients in family meals:

- altering cooking techniques
- reducing portion sizes of richer items
- padding the meal with healthier items.

Altering cooking techniques

- An obvious way to reduce fat is to grill food rather than fry it. It is not simply that grilling avoids putting extra fat into food; it allows some of the fat already within to melt and drip out, whereas frying in oil tends to seal the surface of the food so that more of its own fat is kept inside.

Table 13.2 Fitting savoury foods into the three frequency categories

Celebration or rare treat foods	Weekend foods	Daily basics
Roast with all the trimmings, rich sauces and heaps of stuffing	Simple roast dinner	Oven-baked lean meat with boiled or steamed vegetables
Rich picnic foods such as pork pies, pasties, sausage rolls, samosas, onion bhajis	Special breads with garlic or cheese toppings, white bread, stuffed naan	Wholemeal bread, rolls, sandwiches, herb bread, pitta bread, plain naan
High-fat sandwich fillers such as corned beef, salami, pâté, egg mayonnaise	Canned tuna in oil, premium potato salad or coleslaw*, hummus, full-fat cheese, fish paste	Canned tuna in brine, boiled ham, beef, chicken, cottage cheese, tomato salsa, potato salad or coleslaw with reduced-fat mayonnaise, reduced-fat cheese
Batter-coated foods, deep-fried foods	Sausages, burgers, fish fingers	Grilled lean meat and fish, home-made burgers or nuggets
Quiche, cheese omelette	Spanish omelette	Reduced-fat cheese on toast
Deep-fried chips	Oven chips, roast potatoes	Jacket or boiled potatoes
Steak and kidney pudding*	Lasagne*, shepherd's pie*	Stewed steak with gravy
Crispy cod steaks in batter*	Fish steak in butter sauce*	Baked or poached cod with tomato sauce
Creamy pasta sauces, pesto sauce	Sun-dried tomato sauce	Sieved tomatoes, tomato and herb pasta sauce
Creamy curry sauces* or creamy cook-in sauce*	Tomato-based curries* or cook-in sauces*, vegetable curry*	Stir-fry meat and vegetables

* Refers to standard pre-packaged items rather than home-made varieties or diet-range products.

- Avoid deep-frying anything. Throw out or sell the deep fat fryer and do not be tempted to get another. Deep-frying completely soaks food in oil, leaving it literally dripping fat, which could double its calories.
- Invest in good non-stick pans so that food can be cooked with the bare minimum of oil. This sort of dry-frying or dry-roasting is a good alternative to traditional frying and is easy with a non-stick pan.
- When light- or dry-frying, apply very small amounts of oil using kitchen paper to wipe thinly over the pan's surface (before heating) or invest in an oil sprayer.
- Cook for longer at a lower temperature. If sausages, burgers or other grill items (such as nuggets, or fish in batter or breadcrumbs) are cooked in the top of a hot oven rather than under a grill then the slightly lower temperature will allow more fat to melt out of the meat before the food's surface becomes sealed. They may appear smaller than when fried because more fat will have been lost, but this will leave a higher proportion of nutritious protein behind.
- Reduce the amount of salt added to any foods when cooking. Add herbs and spices to keep food interesting, rather than salt.

- Use alternatives to sugar when preparing sweet things, such as dried or fresh fruit or fruit juice (see below).
- Exchange white flour in recipes for wholemeal flour or oats.
- Steam vegetables (and fish) instead of boiling to improve flavour and texture and to retain vitamins and minerals.

Reduce portion sizes of richer ingredients

Looking at *The Balance of Good Health*, around one-sixth of the daily diet will consist of richer foods with a higher fat or sugar content. Far from being banned, it is just a case of getting the proportions right. Rather than arguing with a reluctant family over how often a favourite food might appear, the alternative approach is to reduce the amount that is served on any occasion so that more frequent appearances will be less of a problem.

- The easiest way to make reductions is to prepare or buy less in the first place, rather than expect people to exercise restraint when food is ready and waiting.
- If large quantities are cheaper or on offer then divide appropriately and freeze in separate bags as soon as purchased. Alternatively, cook it all but put the extra straight into the freezer for an easy meal another day.
- Rather than individual steak and mushroom pies, for example, which tend to have a lot of pastry for the amount of filling, buy one family pie that can be divided up into smaller but juicier portions.
- Stock up on plastic containers with lids, such as old ice-cream cartons, so that leftover food can easily be put in the fridge as soon as it has cooled, rather than be nibbled at the time.
- Try not to let food manufacturers decide on what quantities should be eaten – decide yourself. Watch out for items that are sold in the wrong amount for the family. An example is a packet of eight sausages for a family of five, where one pack in not enough but two packs are too many, or a pack of ten bacon rashers for only three people. Choose an alternative brand or go to the deli-counter or a butcher so that the right quantities can be purchased.

These suggestions will not leave the family hungry because there will be other filling but healthy ingredients on the plate.

Pad meals with healthier ingredients

If families are not used to eating much in the way of fruit and vegetables, then padding out familiar meals is a good way to gradually introduce them. Rather than serving them as a separate portion, virtually all vegetables can be sliced up and added to stews, stir-fries and sauces. Some are best cooked a little first whereas others can be thrown in almost at the last minute. Many can be added uncooked to salads too. Commonplace examples are given in Box 13.1.

Box 13.1 Ideas for adding vegetable padding

Frozen peas, runner beans and broad beans – throw into stir-fries, cook-in sauces, stews and casseroles. They need only a minute or two to heat through and so can be last-minute additions.

Frozen spinach – perfect addition to curries and casseroles, tomato-based pasta sauces or even to parsley sauce.

Peppers, red, yellow or green – can be thrown into stir-fries, or light-fry with onion before adding to casseroles or cook-in sauces. Alternatively, stuff with minced meat and oven bake.

Carrots, swede, turnip, squash – add chunks to casseroles for a slow-cook, but if adding to cook-in sauces that require a shorter cooking time then cut into smaller slices to ensure they cook in time.

Mushrooms – can be added to virtually anything because they need next to no cooking, but can cope with a slow-cook too.

Leeks – go well with onion and can be used instead. Easy padding for slow-cook meals – just throw them in as the liquid is added.

Courgettes – ideal with tomato-based sauces or in stir-fries. Can be dry-fried with garlic and pepper as a delicious alternative.

Broccoli and cauliflower – easy addition to stir-fries and tomato-based sauces. Use small florets to ensure adequate cooking and the stalks can be sliced and added too.

Cabbage – great in stir-fries or light-fried with bacon chunks. Alternatively, use blanched whole leaves to wrap up home-made meat balls, securing the 'parcels' with a wooden cocktail stick.

Marrow – instead of Bolognese sauce with pasta, pour it over a marrow sliced lengthways and hollowed and then bake covered in foil. Serve with pasta or rice.

Sweet corn – tinned sweet corn can be added to soups, stews, stir-fries, salads or sauces, or eaten straight from the tin.

Salad padding – the following can all be added to a plain salad as no cooking is required: peppers, spring onions, thinly sliced courgette, mushroom, broccoli, frozen peas, mangetout or sugar snap peas, sweet corn or baby corn cobs, whole young spinach leaves, grated or thinly sliced carrot, thinly sliced cabbage. To make a salad more substantial, add cold rice, couscous, sliced potato or pasta so that it serves as a main meal.

Meal padding does not have to involve fruit and vegetables. Providing a plate of wholemeal bread or bread sticks alongside the meal is a good way to add more carbohydrate. Beginning with a starter is another way to take the edge off appetite and encourage either carbohydrate or fruit and vegetables to be eaten when appetite is usually at its greatest.

Home-made family favourites such as shepherd's pie can be made very healthy by using lean minced meat or by skimming off fat when the mince is first fried, before adding further ingredients. Many vegetables can be added to the meat for padding too. The potato topping can be mashed using a little light stock and sliced spring onion, rather than extra butter. If pastry pies have been popular, try the same filling but with lightly boiled then sliced potato as a topping instead. Alternatively, use the filling to cover a dish of boiled pasta to create a pasta-bake.

Making 'daily basics' easy

One reason why processed foods have become so popular is because they are quick and easy. With far less teaching of cooking skills in schools nowadays, some families are not confident about cooking traditional dishes and many other parents find they simply do not have enough time.

Daily basics do not always need complex cooking; there are many ways to prepare basic ingredients with just as little effort as putting a pre-packaged tray into an oven or microwave. Some examples are listed in Box 13.2, but many more ideas are available in a wide variety of family cookbooks (*see* Appendix 2).

Box 13.2 Quick and easy daily basics

Jacket potatoes – take five minutes or so in a microwave or a more leisurely hour in the oven.

Boiled potatoes – do not bother peeling them to save time and to retain more nutrients.

Rice – takes around 10–15 minutes to boil. Or try risotto rice (also called Arborio rice) because it is easy to add vegetables, meat and stock during cooking to give a complete meal in itself.

Pasta – try pasta filled with meat or cheese stuffing such as tortellini or cannelloni for a more varied meal.

Couscous – the quickest of convenience foods: just pour boiling water over and wait five minutes! Pre-flavoured varieties are also available or add finely chopped salad or dry-fried vegetables.

Vegetables – try 'ready bags' of mixed vegetables which can be simply heated in the microwave without any preparation at all. Alternatively, invest in a steamer so that vegetables can be easily steamed over other things on the hob.

Pitta bread or tortillas – fill with a quick stir-fry for a change.

Home-made chicken nuggets – make healthy home-made ones with strips of chicken breast brushed with beaten egg or HP sauce and dunked in breadcrumbs. Dry-fry or grill.

Home-made burgers – use lean minced beef, finely chopped onion and a beaten egg and squash into burger shapes. Dry-fry or bake at the top of a hot oven.

Help children move away from a 'junk food' diet

Even though studies have shown that many children enjoy healthy foods, there are many parents who find it difficult to get their children to accept newer, healthier foods and flavours, because they have already developed a strong liking for convenient processed foods.

The family diet can improve without causing upset by introducing change gradually and getting children involved in which healthier options are chosen. Bear in mind the following:

- Try not to cook separate meals for children and adults. If there are twice the meals to cook then convenience foods will be more tempting due to the hassle of so much cooking.
- Use the general rule: if adults wouldn't eat a food because they think it is poor quality, then do not serve it to children either. Convenience foods have their place partly because they can be simple to serve, but also because some taste good. However, many foods designed for children are not only nutritionally poor, but taste awful too. If parents do not like them, do not teach children to develop a liking for them by serving them often.
- To begin with, reduce portion sizes of 'junk' foods and pad with healthier items, rather than reduce how often a food is served, so that children get used to eating healthier foods. Make different food combinations more familiar (for example, sausages with pasta and salad rather than always with chips) before gradually moving towards serving them less often.
- If healthy menus go down well, serve them often.
- Do not worry about the family getting bored with basic foods – people do not grumble about things that are taken for granted. (For example, many adults eat the same breakfast year in, year out from childhood.) People get bored if they are expecting fun but find the reality is less entertaining than expected. They do not get bored when doing routine things that were never likely to give a buzz in the first place. Children are not expecting excitement at every meal, so gourmet dishes are not required on a daily basis.
- Create clear guidelines about when 'junk food' is okay such as 'Junk food is for journeys', when the convenience factor will be useful and an enjoyable rich snack may break up a long stretch in the car.
- Create healthy home-made versions of junk foods such as healthy burgers and chicken nuggets, as above.
- If a child is used to exciting meals, then find varied ways to make meals appealing without resorting to unhealthy ingredients. There are many approaches that can achieve this, such as fascination factors (*see* Chapter 2), ideas for making ordinary meals special (*see* Chapter 10) and variety night meals (below).

Variety night ideas

Novel ideas and themes can introduce just as much interest to a meal as rich foods, and exploring a theme is a good way to get children involved with food (*see* Table 13.3).

Schemes for sugary foods and snacks

Sugary foods are a normal part of most people's diets. The important thing is to make sure they do not make up too big a proportion of the overall diet, leaving little room for healthy ingredients and putting teeth at risk of decay.

For puddings, the same three groups as before can be used to help guide how appropriate they are: celebration or rare treat foods, weekend foods and daily basics. Some examples are given in Table 13.4.

Breakfast cereals can be thought of as either daily basics (unsweetened) or holiday choices (sugar-coated) to give a simple way for children to feel happy

Table 13.3 Themes to help children get involved with food

Theme	Suggestions
Pick a colour night	Get kids to plan different ingredients for, say, red night, or yellow. Blue is probably the trickiest colour to theme a whole meal, but not impossible. Try www.5aday.com for ideas.
Picture plates	Set kids a challenge to make portraits on their plates – suggest useful 'art' ingredients such as spaghetti or peas. Encourage them to eat some of the food first to make room for the picture.
Cook your own tea night	Let children choose the ingredients and teach them how to cook them.
Turf out the cupboards night	It's surprising what is lurking at the back of kitchen cupboards – you might find inspiration or some nasty surprises! Some things, such as dried fruit, can be put in a bowl to be eaten up, or soaked in hot water then added to yoghurt, whereas others will be best reserved for collage material!
Kebab night	Wooden skewers are cheap to buy, and can make roasted vegetables or pieces of meat seem quite different. They're a good idea for barbeques, and fruit kebabs are great too.
Odd combo night	This is a good way to introduce new combinations – why not have steak and strawberries or lamb chops with a dried apricot on top? Kids might dream up any number of funny combinations.
Suits-all soup	If everyone is suggesting a different thing for tea, why not try throwing all the suggestions into one big soup, casserole or dry-roast dish?
Shape night	Similar to pick a colour night, but ingredients must be a certain shape – long and thin, squashy or round. How about star shapes?
Alphabet night	As many ingredients as possible to start with a chosen letter – perhaps a child's name initial.
Build a pizza night	Start with plain pizza bases (available in supermarkets) and let kids experiment with toppings of their choice.
Food from abroad night	Choose a country and explore their dishes – you might try countries your children have learned about at school or places you have visited or would like to visit on holiday.

with unsweetened and ordinary cereals on ordinary days, whilst more sugary varieties are reserved for holidays and perhaps weekends.

Snacks and sweets require a different way of assessing their suitability, because they are eaten so frequently by the majority of children and may form a significant part of the diet. There are three groups: sugar-buzz foods, stodgy sugars and safer sugars, which give an indication of what, if any, useful function they serve within the overall diet.

A high-sugar food will have at least 10 grams of sugars per 100 grams.
A low-sugar food will have less than 2 grams of sugars per 100 grams.

Table 13.4 Fitting sweet foods into the three frequency categories

Celebratory or rare treat foods	Once-weekly or weekend foods	Daily basics
Suet pudding, thick pastry pies with cream	Fruit crumble* with custard, sponge pudding with syrup	Fruit salads, plain and fruit yoghurt, poached pears, fruit compote
Crème brûlée	Fruit cheesecake	Egg custard
Profiteroles, choux buns filled with cream	Lemon meringue pie	Rice pudding
Speciality ice-cream with fudge sauce*	Banana split with chocolate sauce	Plain ice-cream
Festive or novelty cakes with thick icing, butter-cream or fresh cream	Sponge cakes with jam or chocolate filling, carrot cake	Tea breads, fruit scones, Chelsea buns, fruit cake
Bombay mix	Crisps, peanuts	Low-fat crackers and bread sticks

*Refers to standard pre-packaged items rather than home-made varieties or diet-range products.

Sugar-buzz foods

These have a very high sugar content and indeed some are almost entirely sugar, with added colours and flavourings. Most have little filling power, virtually no nutritional value and are fantastic at rotting teeth. Sugary breakfast cereals appear in this group, because many contain over half of their carbohydrate as simple sugars. Even though all cereals are reasonably filling, sugary ones provide far more calories per bowlful, but are no more filling than non-sugared versions.

Sugar-buzz foods may taste nice, but they add very little to a balanced diet and should be eaten sparingly in order not to cause tooth decay.

Stodgy sugars

These sugary foods also contain lots of fat. They may be more filling than sugar-buzz foods, but tend to contain far more calories per mouthful and may be responsible for overweight problems in children. If children like chocolate confectionery and similar stodgy sugars, offer small 'snack-sized' portions and provide a healthy accompaniment such as fruit or a more filling sandwich at the same time, so that appetite can be satisfied without eating too much stodge.

Safer sugars

Sugars in this group have some nutritional value alongside their sweet flavour so that they fit more easily into *The Balance of Good Health*. They may provide vitamins and fibre; they may contain unrefined starchy carbohydrates in addition to the sugar content for slower release of energy; or they may contain dairy products or protein and hence contribute in some way to a balanced diet.

Table 13.5 Examples of sugar-buzz, stodgy sugars and safer sugars foods

Sugar-buzz foods	Stodgy sugars	Safer sugars
Boiled sweets, lollipops, chewy sweets, iced gems	Chocolate confectionery, chocolate-coated biscuits and cakes, plain biscuits	Raisins, nuts, seeds, fruit, cereal bars*, wholemeal scones
Sugar-coated breakfast cereals	Maple and pecan crunchy breakfast cereal, chocolate croissants, pancakes	Sandwiches, toasted tea-cakes, unsweetened cereals such as cornflakes, porridge, muesli
Meringues	Cheesecake, gateaux	Wholemeal fruit crumble and custard, baked apples, carrot cake, fruit muffins, rice pudding
Sorbets, jelly	Speciality ice-creams such as cookie-dough ice cream, or chocolate-coated ice-cream bars	Plain ice-cream, especially with fruit, yoghurt
Fizzy drinks, sports drinks (non-diet)	Milk shakes	Fruit juice, diluted squash, fruit smoothies, semi-skimmed milk

* Applies to lower-sugar versions only as some cereal bars are very high in sugar.

It is worth checking the packaging of any item that claims a health benefit (such as some cereal bars) to make sure it is not awash with added sugar.

Some examples of how foods fit into these categories are given in Table 13.5.

Which snack foods and when?

Wherever possible, choose safer sugars for snacks, which are the most nutritious, particularly when wondering what to put in the snack tin. Keep sugar-buzz foods to a minimum both in terms of portion sizes and frequency. Reserve fizzy or so-called sports drinks for an occasional treat when eating in pubs or restaurants or when there is no easy alternative, because they have significant calorie content and no filling power. They're also terrible for teeth due to their acidity as well as their sugar content. Diet versions are an option, but preferably encourage children to enjoy healthier drinks such as dilute fruit juice, unsweetened tea and coffee, milk and plain water.

If the next meal is a long way off then avoid sugar-buzz foods altogether because they give a rapid rise and fall in blood sugar, which will result in further hunger pangs in a short while. Choose a more filling snack, either from the safer sugars or a combination of a small portion of a stodgy sugar plus the benefit of a safer sugar for filling power.

This is particularly important after taking part in sports, when children tend to feel very hungry. If stodgy sugars are an automatic assumption there is the risk of replenishing far more calories than have just been used up (*see* Chapter 11, p. 126.) A better way to replenish the energy used up in sports is with safer sugars, which tend to be starchy and lower-fat foods, plus plenty of dilute fluids or water, so that blood glucose is maintained without giving the rapid surge and fall that simple sugars give.

Devise household rules for snacks which are easy to stick to, so that children learn to predict what types of food will be suggested when they claim to be 'starving' (*see* Box 13.3). Talking to children about their choice of snacks provides training for later life when older children will be able to take their own money and buy what they want. The more confident they feel about choosing the right thing at the right time, the less likely they will be tempted by inappropriate foods. Although it might be slightly more hassle to prepare slices of toast for hungry youngsters than to open the treat tin, it won't be long before children are old enough to make their own toast, which will give both health and money savings in the long run.

Box 13.3 Healthy snack house rules

- No snacks in the half hour before a meal. (Consider a healthy starter instead.)
- Fruit is always the best choice.
- No snacks during the first hour after a meal. Do not confuse hunger with boredom and try distraction instead of food.
- Do a 'take five' check before choosing rich snacks to see if fruit would be more suitable.
- No snacks or sweet drinks after teeth have been cleaned at night-time.

For serious chocoholics who cannot bear the idea of being deprived of their chocolate 'fix', incorporate something chocolatey into meals, as the dessert, whilst ensuring that the rest of the meal is fairly well balanced. Vary the amount of chocolate and alternatives on offer so children get used to non-chocolate treats without feeling hard done by.

Breakfast reduces snacking later on

Some children refuse to eat breakfast, but tuck into food later in the morning. This first snack is, in effect, a meal and so should fit in with the overall nutritional needs of the day. Once again, if a stodgy snack is the preferred option then add a safer sugar alongside, in order to provide healthy ingredients in addition to fat and sugar.

Studies show children are more likely to eat breakfast if the family sit down together for evening meals and also that breakfast eaters are less likely to be overweight than those who skip it. A starchy start will reduce the likelihood of mid-morning snacking. Breakfast also provides an important opportunity to restock energy reserves that are used up overnight. This may explain why breakfast eaters are more alert mentally. For children who adamantly refuse breakfast, offer a meal replacement bar or a shake fortified with vitamins and minerals mid-morning. A carton of fruit juice or milk would also be preferable to a can of anything fizzy.

Summary points

- Decide whether family foods fit into the daily basics category or whether they would be better kept for weekly treats or reserved for special occasions.
- Modify popular meals that are high in fat or sugar to fit in better with *The Balance of Good Health*.
- Reduce portion sizes of less healthy family favourites or rich treats that appear often.
- Use variety night ideas and fascination factors to make ordinary meals more interesting.
- Choose safe sugars for snacks because they contain some nutritional value, particularly if snacks make up a sizeable portion of the daily diet.
- Encourage children to eat breakfast because it boosts mental alertness in addition to reducing unhealthy snacking later in the morning.

Chapter 14

Vegetarian and vegan eating

This short chapter describes how vegetarian and vegan diets affect nutrition, plus ways to ensure these diets are nutritionally suitable for children.

There are different types of vegetarian diets

Vegetarian eating is commonplace, with many individuals choosing not to eat meat or animal products with varying degrees of strictness. If children follow a restricted diet of any sort then care should be taken to ensure that the essentials of the diet are still available in one form or another.

With due care, vegetarian eating can be a healthy and enjoyable way to eat for both adults and children. Egg and dairy products provide almost all of the nutrients that would otherwise come from meat in the diet, and because there is strong emphasis on wholegrain cereals plus fruit and vegetables, vegetarian diets are usually rich in many useful nutrients.

An American study showed that the diet of vegetarian teenagers contained better amounts of fruit and vegetables and lower amounts of saturated fats than that of meat-eating teenagers, which could well lead to a lower risk of heart disease and cancer if these eating habits continued into adult life.

Vegetarian and vegan eating can be divided into four groups according to their effects on nutrition:

- red meat excluders – eat a normal diet apart from excluding red meat
- permissive vegetarians – avoid all meat, but eat fish in addition to dairy products and eggs
- strict vegetarians – avoid all meat and fish, but eat dairy products and eggs
- vegans – avoid any products that come from animals, including all dairy products and eggs.

As long as the diet still follows the basic outline of *The Balance of Good Health*, with suitable non-meat alternatives, children will have all the nutrients they need. If meat proteins, eggs and dairy products are missing from the diet then far more care is needed to provide suitable replacements for growing children. Figure 14.1 gives an idea of where different essential ingredients of the diet come from and how this fits with different degrees of vegetarian or vegan eating.

Why do people become vegetarian?

There is a variety of reasons why people choose to avoid meat or meat products. These range from compassion for animals; dislike of the taste or texture of meat; peer pressure or a desired sense of independence; concern about food scares or for

	Essential protein	Fibre	Calcium	Iron	Vitamin C	Vitamin B$_{12}$	Vitamin D	Zinc	Folate
Cereals*	+	+++	+	+	/	/	+	+	+
Pulses	+	+++	+	+	/	/	/	/	+
Nuts**	++	++	+	+	/	/	/	/	+
Fruit and veg	+	+	+	+	+++	/	/	/	+++
Seeds	+	++	+	+	/	/	/	/	/
Yeast extract	+	/	/	/	/	++	/	/	++
Infant soya formula	++	/	++	++	+	+	+	+	+
Eggs	+++	/	+	+	/	+	++	/	/
Milk and dairy products	+++	/	+++	/	/	+	++	+	/
Fish	+++	/	++	++	/	++	+++	++	/
White meat	+++	/	/	++	/	++	/	++	/
Red meat	+++	/	/	+++	/	++	/	+++	+

Diet category brackets (left of table, from outermost to innermost): No exclusions to diet; Red meat excluders; Permissive vegetarian diet; Strict vegetarian diet; Vegan diet.

Key and explanatory notes:

/   Nil present or trace only.

+   Small amounts present. Would need to eat large amounts in order to gain enough of the nutrient.

++   Moderate amounts present. Needs to feature in the daily diet in order to provide an adequate supply of the nutrient.

+++   Excellent source of the nutrient.

*   Some cereals are fortified with additional nutrients. Check packaging of individual foods for further details. Lower fibre products are available.

**   If there is a family history of allergies, the introduction of nuts into the diet should be delayed until after the age of 5.

Figure 14.1 Food groups and the essential nutrients they provide.

religious reasons. Children may follow the example of parents, particularly if they understand the issues behind the parents' decisions.

Many youngsters go through phases of disliking meat, which may mirror their growing awareness of farming practices or hearing off-putting information about how processed foods are made. These phases may not last, but care should be taken to make sure the diet is adequate during the phase, because children need good nutrition whilst growing.

Helping children to follow a vegetarian diet successfully

As Figure 14.1 shows, most of the essential nutrients are present in a wide variety of foods and so varied eating is the key to a successful vegetarian diet. Because vegetarian sources of protein are often bulky and contain high fibre, younger children run the risk of filling up before they have taken in enough calories. Also high fibre content can make it harder for the gut to absorb iron and calcium from other foods. To ensure this is not a problem, they should be encouraged to eat plenty of nuts and lower-fibre cereals with not too much reliance on fruit and vegetables. Iron absorption can be improved by including fruit or fruit juice (diluted for babies and children under five) because vitamin C helps absorption.

Ensure that foods containing vitamin B_{12}, such as eggs, yeast extract and fortified breakfast cereals, are included daily.

The diet can be boosted with extra fat to increase the number of calories per mouthful. It is not advised to increase energy intake by providing excess sugar because sugar tends to be nutrient-poor in addition to being linked to tooth decay.

Vegetarian sources of protein tend to contain fewer of the different protein building blocks, or amino acids. To overcome this, combine different sources of proteins together, such as cereals and pulses, so that each source provides a few of the essentials. Examples are baked beans on toast, pitta bread and hummus, lentil stew and rice.

Further advice may be obtained from the Vegetarian Society, www.vegsoc.org. More information about organic food and farming is available at the Henry Doubleday Foundation website, www.hdra.org.uk, or The Soil Association, www.soilassociation.org. Further information about sustainable fish stocks and safe fishing practices can be found at www.fishonline.org.

Vegan eating

Vegan eating takes vegetarianism a stage further, where no animal products are eaten in any form. Humans did not evolve as vegans and so this diet results in nutritional deficiencies unless dietary supplements are taken. In order to comply with vegan principles, fastidious attention to this highly restrictive diet is needed. Because of significant concerns over nutritional deficiencies in vegans, this book does not advise vegan eating for children. The European Prospective Investigation into Cancer and Nutrition study found that 30% of vegans in the UK were severely deficient in vitamin B_{12}, which can lead to permanent nerve damage.

Whilst parents may, by all means, make their children aware of their concerns about farming practices (the main reason why people opt for a vegan diet), young children should be given a diet that fits with *The Balance of Good Health*, which includes some animal food sources in order to be nutritionally complete, with the option of then becoming vegan when they are old enough to make an informed choice.

Many children are highly sensitive to wanting to 'fit in' at school and with friends, making the very limited vegan diet an additional complication in life. If they are gradually introduced to the principles that their parents follow then they may well follow suit as they get older through their own choice, with far less risk of nutritional deficiency than in earlier childhood. Meanwhile, concerned parents should be able to source humanely farmed dairy products, in order to put their own children's health first, when it matters most.

If families feel they would like to bring up their children to follow vegan principles, nutritional advice from a registered dietician or nutritionist is strongly recommended. Further information is available through the Vegan Society, www.vegansociety.com.

Summary points

- The key to a successful vegetarian diet is varied eating, in order that the full array of essential nutrients is included in the diet.
- Children eating a vegetarian diet should steer away from too much fibre, because it can fill them up before enough calories have been eaten and may reduce the absorption of iron and calcium.
- Vegan eating is not recommended for children due to the risk of vitamin B_{12} deficiency.

Chapter 15

An A to Z of conditions that affect eating and weight in younger children

This chapter looks at a variety of conditions that have an effect on either a child's weight, eating tendency or ability to exercise, with details of how and when to obtain further advice. Whilst some conditions can safely be treated at home, other conditions require professional help, which can usually be obtained through the family doctor or health visitor. This chapter is not intended to replace the need for a medical opinion, but aims to help with deciding when to seek advice. When in doubt, it is always better to ask sooner rather than later.

- Abdominal pain
- Allergies to food
- Anorexia or loss of appetite
- Appendicitis
- Asthma
- Coeliac disease or wheat sensitivity
- Constipation
- Cow's milk or lactose intolerance
- Cystic fibrosis
- Depression
- Diabetes
- Diarrhoea
- Gastro-oesophageal reflux
- Inflammatory conditions of the gut
- Phenylketonuria
- Pyloric stenosis
- Thyroid disorders
- Tooth decay
- Worms

Abdominal pain

Abdominal pain is one of the commonest ailments in childhood; along with coughs and colds it features daily in every doctor's surgery. It is not an illness in itself, but a symptom. Sometimes there is an obvious cause, such as constipation or appendicitis (see below), but at other times no cause can be found. When assessing a child, the first question to ask is whether it is a new problem or if it has been grumbling on for some time.

If a child has become unwell quite rapidly, with vomiting, a temperature and abdominal pains, especially if the pain is worse on moving, then prompt advice should be sought either from a family doctor or a health helpline such as NHS Direct (*see* Appendix 2), who can discuss the child's symptoms and advise on how quickly to seek further help.

If a child has had milder intermittent tummy ache then symptoms could be improved without the need to see a doctor by trying simple measures, as outlined below. If the symptoms persist, however, it makes sense to seek further advice.

Colic

Our guts do not sense things in the same way that skin does – the gut is not sensitive to touch or temperature, but it is very sensitive to being stretched or to griping, for example when it is stretched by trapped wind or a hard motion, or if it clamps down in spasm. This causes a pain called *colic*, which usually comes in nasty waves that build up gradually, become a tight gripping pain and then slowly ease off again. A person with colic tends to writhe around, finding it difficult to get comfortable.

Colic may be caused by a variety of things; constipation is by far the commonest cause, but it will accompany diarrhoea and sickness bugs, and sometimes seems to happen for no apparent reason. The section on constipation looks at ideas on how to treat colicky tummy pains.

Abdominal migraine

This is a term sometimes used to describe intermittent tummy pains that leave a child feeling under the weather for a few hours but then subside as oddly as they arrived. There is nothing to suggest spasm of the gut as a cause, as in colic, and no other signs to suggest a urine infection or appendicitis. The pain may be accompanied by a headache; indeed, as time goes by, some children find the headaches become more troublesome with each bout but the tummy pain gets less, so that by adulthood they simply suffer migraine headaches. A family doctor will have some suggestions on how to treat this condition, and happily many children gradually grow out of the phase.

Swollen abdominal glands

Another fairly common condition is where the glands in the tummy become inflamed – a condition impressively called mesenteric adenitis. In the same way that glands in the neck become tender and swollen when they are fighting infections, the glands in the abdomen can do the same. A child with this condition will often have tender glands in the neck, symptoms of a viral infection such as a cough, cold or sore throat, and may have a slight temperature. Simple measures, such as regular paracetamol, plenty of clear fluids and some fresh air, are all that are required to keep a child comfortable whilst their immune system gets on with the business in hand – fighting infection. Most viral infections will last anything from a week to a fortnight, and so the abdominal pains may grumble on throughout this time. If there is concern then a family doctor will check the child over, but do not expect antibiotics as they have no effect against viral infections.

Urine infection

In older children, a urine infection usually causes the typical symptoms of pain or discomfort whilst passing urine plus a feeling of urgency and wanting to pass small amounts of urine very frequently. Younger children, however, will often become generally unwell, with abdominal pain, vomiting, a high temperature or even rigors – when the body shakes uncontrollably as temperature rises and falls. Children who have been out of nappies may start to have accidents or wet the bed, or may simply be clingy, off food and out of sorts. If there is doubt about the cause of a child's illness, taking a specimen of urine along to the doctor's appointment may provide the answer.

If a child is found to have a urine infection, it is quite likely that, in addition to prescribing antibiotics, the doctor will arrange some further tests, such as an ultrasound scan of the child's kidneys and bladder.

Allergies to food

Allergies are becoming increasingly common and may arise at any time of life, particularly in childhood. If a child has a suspected food allergy, seek advice from a doctor or a registered dietician so that the condition can be diagnosed correctly, rather than simply excluding the suspected food. This will ensure that no dietary deficiency results from avoiding the problem food, and will provide the opportunity to learn what to do if a child accidentally comes into contact with the problem food in future.

Most people who are allergic will suffer mild irritating symptoms, but occasionally, in severe allergy, a person can suffer an acute and sometimes life-threatening reaction called *anaphylaxis*. This is an emergency situation where the body reacts rapidly, causing swelling of the mouth and throat, which results in breathing difficulties and can cause collapse. It requires immediate help and an ambulance should be summoned if suspected. If a person has suffered an anaphylactic reaction, it is wise to wear a Medic-Alert bracelet and to consider carrying an emergency supply of adrenaline. This should be discussed with a doctor.

Box 15.1 lists common foods that can trigger allergic reactions. Certain foods, for example milk, wheat, eggs and nuts, cause more of a problem than others because they may be hidden in many basic foods, making them hard to avoid.

Box 15.1 Common foods that can trigger allergic reactions

- Seafood, especially prawns and mussels
- Peanuts
- Eggs
- Milk
- Wheat
- Citrus fruits and strawberries
- Soya products
- Bananas
- Food additives
- Chocolate

There is currently no cure for food allergies, which means the food must be avoided in order to prevent the symptoms it triggers. Mild reactions can be improved by the use of antihistamine tablets, but it is preferable to avoid the allergen in case repeated exposure escalates a mild reaction into a more severe one. Common symptoms from any food allergy are similar to those described for peanut or milk allergy below.

Peanut allergy

Peanut allergy is unfortunately becoming more common, although it is not clear exactly why. Anyone can develop it, even in later life, but it is commoner in people who have atopic (meaning allergy-related) conditions such as asthma, eczema or hay fever. These sometimes run in families (atopic families) and can be inherited.

Because there is a chance that eating peanuts in pregnancy and during breast-feeding may increase the risk of a child developing peanut allergy, the Department of Health recommends that a mother from an atopic family should avoid peanuts during this time. Children from such families should avoid peanuts and peanut products until they are at least three years old.

If allergic to peanuts there is a high chance of being allergic to other nuts too, such as walnuts, cashews or brazil nuts, and sometimes to hazelnuts, pine nuts and pistachios, so these are best avoided too.

What happens if a sufferer comes into contact with peanuts?

There can be two main reactions: a mild reaction or severe anaphylactic reaction. In mild peanut allergy, varying symptoms come on quickly, with perhaps an itchy rash, tingling of the mouth, diarrhoea or sickness. In severe cases, the person may have facial swelling, difficulty breathing and even collapse. Both mild and severe reactions can happen up to six hours after eating peanuts, and even if only tiny traces of peanut have been consumed.

Peanut allergy is now well recognised and food manufacturers have improved the labelling of many foods to inform if peanut traces are present. Look for 'not suitable for nut allergy sufferers' or 'may contain nuts' as a guide, although some manufacturers have taken this too far and are labelling all their products so as to avoid liability.

Because there is no cure to the underlying allergy, an affected person needs to avoid any contact with peanut products. In particular, check the ingredient list of:

- baked foods, such as cakes and biscuits
- cereals
- oriental dishes
- ice-creams
- health bars
- pastry
- savoury snacks.

Some restaurants are following suit with clear labelling on menus, but others are happy to advise on particular dishes if asked.

Box 15.2 details what a person should do if they witness someone having a reaction to nuts.

Box 15.2 Action points if a person is found reacting to nuts

- Remove any nuts from the person immediately.
- Ask for immediate assistance. Call 999 for an ambulance if the reaction is rapid or severe, with collapse, facial swelling or difficulty breathing.
- Do your best to keep calm and to reassure the person that help is being arranged.
- For a mild reaction you might contact the person's GP, the casualty department, or use the NHS advice line, NHS Direct, on 0845 4647 for further guidance on what to do.

With a degree of care and caution, a person with peanut allergy can live a perfectly normal life. About 25% of children affected will grow out of their allergy, and others will suffer milder reactions as they get older. Consider wearing a Medic-Alert bracelet or necklace and make sure that schools, nurseries and clubs are informed about the condition. More information and advice on treatment is available from the Great Ormond Street Family Resource Centre: 020 7813 8558, or on various websites (*see* Appendix 2).

Milk allergy

Allergy to cow's milk is the most common food allergy in children. Whilst rarely it may be serious, it more commonly causes a mild reaction, which many children grow out of by the age of three.

Milk allergy is a separate condition from lactose (or cow's milk) intolerance, which is described further on. It arises when a person's immune system reacts against the proteins in milk, seeing them as harmful and resulting in one or more hypersensitivity reactions (*see* Box 15.3).

Box 15.3 Hypersensitivity reactions from milk allergy

- Skin reactions – rashes, hives, eczema and swelling of the mouth
- Effects on the gut – diarrhoea, bloating, vomiting, cramps
- Effects on the airways – runny nose, sneezing, itchy or watery eyes, wheeze and cough
- Anaphylaxis (rare effect) – breathing difficulty, facial swelling or collapse

---

If a baby is allergic to cow's milk, it is likely they will also be allergic to the milk protein in goat's or sheep's milk, or even to the proteins in soya formula. There are some highly hydrolysed milk formulas suitable for babies with cow's milk allergy, but it is essential to seek medical advice when deciding how to proceed. Because there is no cure for milk allergy, the only way to avoid it is to cut out milk from the diet.

Milk is a common ingredient in many foods and may be listed under strange names on the ingredients panel (*see* Box 15.4).

Box 15.4 Some alternative names for milk products

- Butter solids/fat
- Casein or caseinate, hydrolysed casein or sodium caseinate
- Whey or delactosed or demineralised whey, or whey protein concentrate
- Dried milk or dry milk solids or milk derivative
- Lactalbumin
- Lactate or lactose
- Lactoferrin
- Lactoglobulin
- Rennet casein
- Sour cream solids
- Sour milk solids

Because milk is such a good source of protein, calcium and vitamins A and B, it is essential to find suitable replacements if it has to be excluded from a child's diet. Non-dairy protein can be found in meat, fish, soya and some green vegetables. Non-dairy calcium is found in sardines, watercress, nuts, figs and rhubarb. Vitamins will be found in fruit and vegetables (especially carrots for vitamin A) and in fortified cereals, fish, seeds and nuts.

It can be hard work excluding milk entirely from a child's diet, but there are many products now available in supermarkets to make the task a little easier. Table 15.1 lists some milk product substitutes. Be wary of soya products if there is a chance that the child is allergic to soya protein too. Discuss this with a doctor or dietician before choosing soya alternatives.

Egg allergy

Egg allergy is significant not only because egg is hidden in many foods, especially cakes, biscuits, pastries, some breads and many sauces, but it is also used in the manufacture of some vaccines. If a child is allergic to egg, remind a doctor or nurse about egg allergy before vaccinations or injections. Check the ingredients

Table 15.1 Ideas for substitution of milk products

Milk product	Non-dairy substitute
Milk	Soya, rice milk, oat milk, coconut milk, nut milk
Butter/margarine	Pure oil margarines, soya spread
Yoghurt	Soya yoghurt, oat yoghurt
Cheese	Rice cheese, soya cheese
Cream	Soya cream, coconut cream
Ice-cream	Rice ice-cream, soya ice-cream
Chocolate	Carob, vegan chocolates

list of foods carefully and look out for the various alternative names that egg may be listed as (*see* Box 15.5).

Box 15.5 Some alternative names for egg derivatives

- Albumin
- Egg protein, powder, white or yolk
- Dried, frozen or pasteurised egg
- Globulin
- Livetin
- Ovalbumin
- Ovaglobulin
- Ovomucin
- Ovovitellin or vitellin
- Lecithin (also known as E322) may be derived from eggs, although it is more often derived from soya. This is usually clarified on an ingredients list.

Anorexia or loss of appetite

Anorexia means loss of appetite and is a separate thing from the condition anorexia nervosa, which is covered in the companion book *Weight Matters for Young People*.

Many things will cause appetite to tail off, especially infections such as coughs and colds, urine infection or appendicitis. If a child has a cough, cold or sickness and diarrhoeal bug, loss of appetite is expected to some extent. As long as the child is taking enough fluids and is passing urine several times throughout each day, short-term loss of appetite is not a problem. Even skinny children can tolerate not eating for a few days without coming to any harm, as long as they keep drinking.

If appetite fails to return after a few days, consider seeking advice from a doctor.

Another reason for appetite to disappear is worry and sadness. Many children as well as adults will lose their appetite in times of stress, so if there are no obvious reasons for a usually healthy child to be off their food, then consider emotional problems as a possible cause. New situations such as a change in school, or emotional upheaval such as parental divorce, will frequently be accompanied by a change in appetite. In older children, drug use may take away appetite and is sometimes associated with weight loss and change in behaviour or personality.

Remember that following a growth spurt, a child who usually has a good appetite may go through a phase of eating very little, simply because energy requirements have tailed off. This is normal and, as long as they are used to eating according to their natural appetite, they will regulate the amount they eat without needing to think about it. When they need more energy they will begin to eat more again.

Following a prolonged illness where a child may have lost weight, appetite can be slow to recover, sometimes because the sight of food reminds the child about the illness itself, but also because we get used to eating less. In this situation, the balance of foods eaten is just as important as ever – a recuperating child will need plenty of vitamins, minerals, fibre and protein to enable healthy growth to begin again. Rather than piling large amounts of food on the plate, offer foods that are more energy-dense, such as full-fat dairy products, creamy sauces and fried rather than grilled meat or fish, to increase the amount of calories eaten without having to eat large quantities. Plain foods are more likely to be acceptable than heavily spiced or strong flavoured foods. If nausea remains a problem, try small amounts of bland foods that have little smell, such as tinned fruit, milk puddings and breakfast cereals. Once a child gets used to eating more varied foods again, appetite will improve.

Appendicitis

This is the commonest reason for emergency surgery in children. It is sometimes easy to diagnose, but at other times can be a real puzzle because the usual symptoms are not always obvious.

The appendix is a small, blind-ended part of the gut, attached near to where the small and the large bowel join together in the bottom right-hand corner of the tummy. If it gets blocked then infection can seep through the walls of the appendix, which can even burst. The resulting inflammation, known as peritonitis, can make a child extremely ill, so any suspicion of appendicitis must be carefully assessed and the appendix may be removed even when it is healthy if abdominal pain is not settling.

Appendicitis usually starts with vague tummy ache and loss of appetite. The pain soon moves down into the bottom right corner and may be accompanied by a slight temperature, vomiting and reluctance to move due to this worsening the pain. Younger children, however, may not show any of the usual symptoms, but just appear unwell. Abdominal pain with loss of appetite should always be checked out. If a child has a hearty appetite but has some abdominal pain, it is less likely to be appendicitis.

Once the appendix becomes inflamed it does not usually settle on its own, it simply gets worse until it is removed by performing a small surgical operation. If in doubt, always seek help as this condition can worsen quickly, especially in very young children.

Asthma

Whilst asthma is a condition of the lungs, it is included in this book on weight and eating because of its effect on a child's ability to exercise, which can have an enormous impact on weight. Asthma is now a very common childhood ailment, affecting at least one in ten children, and is still on the increase. Because it can sometimes be serious, many parents feel anxious about their asthmatic child and some may find themselves being overprotective. If a child senses this it can reduce their confidence in dealing with asthma symptoms, so that tolerance of exercise and general fitness are likely to suffer. Boost an asthmatic child's confidence by looking at the following aspects and encourage them to join in along with everyone else:

- If an asthmatic child is prone to coughing when taking part in games, then improved asthma control might help. This may involve changing the type of inhaler or increasing the dose of existing ones – a family doctor or asthma nurse will advise on this.

- Keep a 'reliever' inhaler to hand during and after games and following break time, particularly during cold weather.
- Challenge school rules if they insist that all medication needs to be kept in a locked cupboard. Reliever inhalers (which are very safe even in the wrong hands) are far more use in pockets or sports bags than locked in a school cupboard. Most children would rather miss out on treatment and cough quietly than be seen making frequent trips to the school office.
- Avoid excuses for missing games and PE, and encourage plenty of physical hobbies because asthmatic children need to keep fit just as much as other children.
- Make sure an asthmatic child knows what to do if they feel breathless, and inform school and clubs about their condition.

Coeliac disease or wheat sensitivity

Coeliac disease is a condition where a food protein called gluten reacts with the lining of the small bowel. Gluten is found in wheat, barley, rye, and to a lesser extent oats. The body's immune system starts to think the small bowel lining is foreign and so attacks it, so that it can no longer absorb nutrients and vitamins properly. In particular, if coeliac disease is left untreated it causes difficulty in absorbing iron and folic acid, causing anaemia; calcium, which can lead to weaker bones and ultimately osteoporosis; and calories in general because the surface area of the gut is reduced, leading to weight loss or failure to thrive.

The diagnosis of coeliac disease is made by a specialist (such as a gastroenterologist or paediatrician) and usually involves blood tests and a biopsy of the small bowel, done under mild sedation. A positive blood test for anti-endomysial antibodies usually indicates coeliac disease is present, but a negative test does not rule it out, so biopsy is usually necessary too. A gluten-free diet should not be started without medical advice, especially if diagnostic tests are planned, or else signs of the disease may disappear before it has been confirmed.

It is important to confirm the diagnosis to avoid potentially serious complications if it is left untreated, including an increased risk of cancer. This risk shrinks if the disease is kept at bay by sticking to a gluten-free diet. In addition, because a gluten-free diet requires commitment and understanding, it is not a diet to be tried on the off chance.

The gluten-free diet

Many foods are naturally gluten-free, such as fruit and vegetables, fresh meat, fish, cheese, eggs and milk, because they do not contain any wheat, rye, barley or oats.

Foods that contain flour, such as bread, cakes, pastries, biscuits and puddings, should all be avoided, but there are many hidden sources of gluten to avoid too. In processed foods, flour may used for binding ingredients, in fillings or as a carrier for flavourings and will not always be listed on the ingredients panel if only a small amount is contained.

Oats, whilst being low in gluten, are not entirely gluten-free, especially if milled or processed alongside other grains. There is some evidence that mild coeliac sufferers can tolerate small amounts of oats (up to 50 grams per day), but someone with more troublesome symptoms should avoid oats in addition to other cereals. This is best discussed with a specialist.

In addition, wheat or wheat flour can contaminate other usually gluten-free products if they are processed or manufactured in the same place.

The Coeliac Society, www.coeliac.co.uk, provides a full listing of all gluten-free products, which is regularly updated. There is a variety of specially manufactured wheat starch foods that comply with the International Gluten-free Standard and so are suitable for a gluten-free diet. In the UK these foods are available on prescription through a family doctor.

Constipation

It is not how often a motion is passed that counts, rather that the process works easily and with no straining or discomfort. As a general rule, people who go regularly to the toilet are less prone to constipation than those people who go infrequently. There is a huge variation in 'normal' – some people go at least once or twice a day, but for others it may be a weekly drama associated with cramps, nausea and even blood in the motion.

If a child is straining to pass a motion and goes less than three or four times a week, it is likely that they are short of fibre in the diet. If this pattern continues into adulthood, there will be an increased risk of piles, diverticular disease and even bowel cancer, and so it is worth sorting this out at the earliest opportunity and learning a healthy approach to fibre in the diet.

Colic is common if the diet is low in fibre, because the gut has to work hard in order for motions to pass along. Eating more fibre and fruit and vegetables helps to 'bulk up' the motion, so that it can travel more smoothly through the gut with less griping.

In addition, encouraging plenty of fluids and exercise will help the gut to work more smoothly.

Particularly for very young children, it is important to get the balance of fibre right, because too much fibre may cause diarrhoea and colicky tummy pains. Some foods can trigger loose motions, whereas other sources of fibre may suit well. Try a variety of things to see if there are certain basic foods, such as wholemeal bread, higher-fibre breakfast cereals, and some fruits and vegetables, that reliably keep the bowel working smoothly and so should feature as daily basic foods. There is no reason why a tablespoon of the reliable higher-fibre ingredient can't be mixed with a whole variety of other lower-fibre foods if it tastes better that way. See Chapter 12 for more ideas on high-fibre foods.

Cow's milk or lactose intolerance

Cow's milk or lactose intolerance is a separate condition from cow's milk allergy, which is covered on page 175. Lactose is the main sugar found in milk and is digested in the body by an enzyme called lactase. In lactose intolerance, this enzyme is in short supply or even absent altogether, resulting in an inability to digest milk. Lactose intolerance is a common condition and is not life-threatening. Its prevalence in the UK is estimated to be about 5%.

The amount of lactase that humans produce tails off after the age of two, although in the west many adults produce enough lactase to be able to digest milk. However, in some parts of the world, such as Asia and Africa, up to 90% of people are lactose intolerant. This is not a problem because milk does not traditionally form part of the typical adult diet in these regions.

Lactose intolerance causes nausea, cramps, bloating, wind and diarrhoea. These symptoms may come on soon after drinking milk, but may also happen many hours later. If a person produces small amounts of lactase, they may be able to tolerate small amounts of milk and only get symptoms if a lot of milk is consumed.

Diagnosis of lactose intolerance can be done by several tests, depending on the age of the child. For older children, the hydrogen breath test may be performed. Following a milk drink, the breath is monitored for the presence of hydrogen, which is a by-product of fermented lactose in the gut. Because this test requires the child to drink milk, which may trigger a bout of diarrhoea, it is not suitable for small children or babies, who may suffer unacceptable dehydration from this test. For younger children a simple stool sample can be checked for reducing substances and pH, which may be sufficient to show lactose intolerance, although it is not as sensitive a test. For babies, many paediatricians are happy to recommend a trial of a milk-free diet, using an approved soya formula as a replacement, to see if this clears up the problem, rather than having them undergo any tests.

Cystic fibrosis

Cystic fibrosis is a genetic disease which interferes with mucus-secreting glands in the body. These are found mainly in the lungs, the pancreas and the sweat glands of the skin. Cystic fibrosis causes chronic cough and chest infection and problems with food digestion, because the lungs and pancreas gland become clogged with thick sticky mucus. The skin also loses excessive salt in the sweat.

The disease is usually discovered in early childhood because of poor weight gain, chronic cough or loose, offensive motions, due to fat remaining undigested as it passes through the gut. It is an uncommon condition. It requires specialist treatment and follow-up and there are now many treatments that can help a sufferer to get on with life, although there is as yet no cure. Treatment involves taking pancreatic enzyme supplements, topping up vitamin intake and eating as high a calorie diet as a child can manage. This usually means smaller but more frequent meals and plenty of snacks in between.

A specialist treatment centre will provide advice and support from a dietician. Chest infections must be treated very promptly and most sufferers need to do daily physiotherapy in order to keep things under control.

Because children with cystic fibrosis have to eat plenty of sugary foods to keep their energy intake up, they must take extra care of their teeth. This involves:

- brushing teeth at least twice a day after meals, using a small amount of fluoride toothpaste
- rinsing the mouth with water after sugary snacks or drinks
- regular dental checks, at least every four months.

If there are any concerns that a child could have cystic fibrosis, a family doctor will be able to decide if further investigations are appropriate.

Depression

Although there is a tendency to think of depression as an adult condition, it can affect children too. One problem is that it is not easy to diagnose – many children have fluctuating episodes of unhappiness, even well-adjusted, straightforward children. But at the other end of the spectrum, some children have sad, challenging home circumstances that would produce low mood in anybody. The distinction between going through a sad phase and actually suffering depression is still up for debate, but it is clear that some children can be helped by seeing their sadness and despair as an illness, rather than as a 'bad mood' that should have passed off with a quick hug or a walk in the park.

What does depression feel like, and what has it to do with weight and eating?

Unless you have had depression, it is hard to imagine why the sufferer can't just pull their socks up and put a brave face on things. But shaking off depression is not the same as trying to cheer up after losing a football match. It is an illness and a surprisingly physical one too (*see* Box 15.6).

Box 15.6 Physical symptoms of depression

- Headaches
- Backache
- Tiredness and physical exhaustion
- Nausea and loss of appetite, leading to weight loss, or
- Excessive hunger, leading to binge eating and weight gain
- Abdominal gripes and diarrhoea
- Anxiety symptoms such as breathlessness, pins and needles and panic attack
- Blurred vision
- Tremor
- Hot flushes and mood swings

In addition to feeling sad, tearful and as though there is no light at the end of the tunnel, many people with depression feel that there is something physically wrong with them. Sometimes fear of an illness can be a reason why depression develops in the first place, and then the physical symptoms that depression brings make the sufferer quite convinced that the illness must be a reality. This can make it hard to accept that the real underlying problem is depression, but talking about these symptoms with a doctor can help to put the jigsaw together.

In younger children who are not grown up enough to express how they feel or recognise that they are unhappy, depression may appear as behaviour problems, such as temper tantrums, an inability to get started with a task, school refusal, withdrawn behaviour or aggressive or destructive tendencies.

A central problem with depression is loss of self-esteem so that the sufferer feels worthless and like a failure. They no longer feel able to face problems, feel a burden to other people and lack confidence in their abilities, thoughts and in other people.

Depression may come as a reaction to being in a difficult situation, such as being bullied, or there may be no obvious reason for confidence to vanish and for depression to occur – it just happens.

It is not only because depression can cause weight and appetite to fluctuate that it is included in this book: depression is very significant with regard to eating disorders, which are covered in the companion book *Weight Matters for Young People*.

How may a parent tell the difference between sadness and depression?

The main factor that distinguishes depression is the time-scale. Depression is not an occasional bad mood; it persists for weeks or, more usually, months, and occasionally years. It can be seen as a spectrum of symptoms, ranging from low moods, tearfulness and loss of interest at the milder end to suicidal thoughts and attempts to self-harm at the other.

Children do not usually show the classical symptoms of depression that are found in adults – those of weight loss, sleep disturbance and strong feelings of guilt. Instead, a child with depression is more likely to be irritable, complain of headaches, run away from home, play truant or show a decline in schoolwork. These symptoms may also make a parent question whether their child has begun to experiment with drugs, because drug use can result in similar changes in a child's outlook and mood. The fact that drug use can bring about depression and vice versa makes it harder still to understand what problems a child may be facing. Drug use will usually give other clues that depression alone wouldn't produce, such as a change in friends or problems with stealing in order to pay for drugs.

If symptoms have become persistent then it is advisable to discuss this with a family doctor. It is not a parent's job to diagnose the condition, rather to help their child to find help if struggling with problems that won't go away.

How can a child with depression be helped?

A problem shared is a problem halved.

Talking about problems is a very valuable way to help anyone with depression. From a child's view, life will feel very complicated if faced with grown-up problems, such as having to care for a disabled parent or being targeted by someone who is pushing drugs, when the child's own experiences of how to deal with it are limited. Family support is less available nowadays because in many households both parents work or they may live separately, so that children do not get as much opportunity to share their feelings and problems. They may be more likely to seek guidance from equally young and inexperienced friends, read advice on the internet or in magazines, or follow celebrity role models than to ask a family member.

Putting time aside to share simple things with a depressed child may be a good way to show that a parent wants to listen and to help, whereas announcing a five-minute slot within which all issues must be done and dusted is likely to confirm the child's view that he doesn't count. In families that are not used to sharing emotional worries, it can take a bit of practice to 'open up' and the youngster may need reassurance that the person listening to their worries won't think they are silly or being pathetic. Children are often surprised to hear that grown-ups also worry about silly things or may struggle to deal with problems.

It will help children to learn that having an emotional reaction to a problem is normal. Getting upset after a disaster is perfectly reasonable and is something we all need to work through. It is not unreasonable to get angry about things, but it is essential to learn positive ways to deal with that anger and to put things in perspective. Show children how they can cope better and improve many symptoms by using simple measures:

- Sleep will be improved by exercise earlier in the day and by fewer drinks late at night.
- Stopping watching scary films or playing violent computer games may allow nightmares to fade away. Go for sports-related action entertainment if a child demands a buzz. Check the age rating on videos and games if unsure what is appropriate for the age of the child.
- Hiding the alarm clock will stop the irritation of clock watching in the small hours.
- Organising tasks to fill empty hours may give the day more structure and make it feel more manageable.
- Setting simple tasks that are easily achievable, such as making the bed or taking a daily shower, will generate both a sense of achievement and the start of feeling in control of life.
- Aggression can be eased by a physical workout – hitting a punch bag or kicking a ball.
- Positive thoughts can be practised – 'Is your glass half empty or is it half full?'
- Big problems can usually be broken down into smaller ones that are easier to tackle bit by bit – 'One step at a time.'
- There is no point worrying too much about potential problems that have not yet arrived – 'Cross that bridge when you get to it.'

Counselling is an effective approach, although there is sometimes a problem gaining access to a counselling service because of long waiting lists. A family doctor can refer a child to the local child psychology services if a family is worried.

Unlike in adulthood, where antidepressant medication has been tried and tested and found to be beneficial, antidepressant use in children is controversial. Many studies have found very little benefit in giving antidepressants to children and some studies have shown worsening symptoms such that some antidepressants are no longer recommended in people under 18. However, they may be used in severe depression, where the benefits are more likely to outweigh the risks.

What is the risk of suicide in a child with depression?

Suicide is rare in younger children and it is not strongly linked to depression. Suicidal attempts are more often related to aggression and use of alcohol or drugs, which can make a person react unpredictably and out of character.

Never brush off a young person's remarks if they include ideas of self-harm, regardless of whether their low mood is a new problem or something that has cropped up before; seek advice promptly from your doctor or casualty department, or try phoning a support service such as The Samaritans (08457 909090), or see their website www.samaritans.org.uk or email them at Jo@samaritans.org. Alternatively, look in the *Yellow Pages* for a local phone number as they have over 200 local support offices.

Happily, there has been a reduction in the rate of suicide since the change in law regarding the sale of paracetamol in the UK, so that only small quantities can be sold. Despite wide scepticism amongst the general public about this legislation, it has been shown to be helpful. Making large quantities of tablets less easy to obtain – which includes keeping only limited supplies in the home too – will reduce the chance of both accidental and planned self-poisoning.

Diabetes

Diabetes (or diabetes mellitus, as it is sometimes called) occurs when blood sugar (glucose) is higher than normal. There are two main types: type 1 diabetes and type 2 diabetes.

Type 1 diabetes usually develops in children or young adults and is also known as juvenile or insulin-dependent diabetes. It is not uncommon, occurring in around one in 250 people. The problem occurs because the body stops producing insulin – which is the hormone that regulates blood sugar – and so blood sugar levels creep up and up until the person becomes very unwell.

It comes on quickly over days or weeks and common symptoms include thirst, passing a lot of urine, tiredness, weight loss and feeling unwell. If it is left untreated, the person will become dehydrated and may lapse into a coma or even die. The condition requires treatment for life with daily insulin injections to replace the insulin that the body no longer produces.

Type 2 diabetes is usually a condition of later life, although it is strongly linked to obesity. Because obesity is now very common and is affecting more and more children, this has led to cases of type 2 diabetes being found in childhood too. It is also called late-onset diabetes or non-insulin dependent or diet-controlled diabetes. The problem is that even though the body continues to produce insulin, it does not produce enough and the cells of the body are unable to use what is there. This is called 'insulin resistance' and causes blood sugar to gradually creep up, but this usually comes on more slowly than in type 1 diabetes.

Symptoms include thirst, passing a lot of urine, tiredness, weight loss and feeling generally unwell, just as in type 1 diabetes, but many people actually have no symptoms and the condition may go unnoticed for some time.

Both types can be detected by a simple 'dipstick' test on a urine specimen and will be confirmed on a blood sample. Further information is available through the British Diabetic Association, now known as Diabetes UK, www.diabetes.org.uk.

What problems does diabetes cause?

If diabetes is untreated or poorly controlled it causes problems both in the short and the long term.

Short-term problems

- When sugar levels rise, it causes the body to produce more urine, causing thirst, dehydration and the need to pass more urine, especially at night. This can lead to drowsiness and a serious illness called ketosis, but it is very treatable if prompt help is sought.

- Some people think that if a person has an illness that puts them off their food, such as flu or a stomach bug, they will need less insulin because they are not eating. In fact the opposite is usually true – an illness will make blood sugar rise and so insulin often needs to be increased if one occurs. If a diabetic person feels unwell for any reason, it is important to check sugar levels more frequently and adjust insulin accordingly.
- Too much insulin can cause problems too: if sugar levels drop too low, which is called hypoglycaemia, a person will feel sweaty, confused, unwell and may lose consciousness. This can be treated by giving sugar in the form of sweets, a sugary drink or an injection of glucagon – a hormone that has the opposite effect to insulin. Some young children have been saviours to their diabetic parent by knowing that if their parent becomes drowsy they should pop a sweet in their mouth and call for help.

Long-term problems

It is very important for any diabetic person to keep their sugar levels as well controlled as possible because good control reduces the chance of long-term diabetic problems.

Too much sugar in the bloodstream is a bit like having 'dirty' blood rather than 'clean' blood circulating. Picture a hosepipe: if dirty water runs through it, eventually some of the dirt sticks to the walls and clogs it up so that less water can pass through. It is exactly the same with diabetes: high sugar levels make blood vessel walls become clogged up with something called 'atheroma' and this causes hardening as well as narrowing of the arteries. This can mean that some organs in the body become short of blood and oxygen, causing heart attacks, stroke and problems with circulation in the legs. It can also damage the kidneys and some nerves and create problems with vision.

However, atheroma is not only caused by diabetes: other problems that clog up blood vessels include a high cholesterol level, high blood pressure, smoking and getting too little exercise. Aiming to keep fit and healthy, keep weight under control and not to smoke are all very important aspects for someone with diabetes, because all these measures will help to keep their blood a bit 'cleaner' and reduce the chance of diabetic-related conditions.

How is diabetes controlled?

There are three main aims for treatment of a diabetic:

1 The first is to control blood sugar as carefully as possible. Type 1 diabetes requires lifelong daily insulin, which is given by injection because it cannot be absorbed through the gut. After diagnosis, a newly diabetic person will have tuition in how to measure their blood sugar and give themselves injections. This can be hard to accept for some people, but support is available for those who are having difficulties. Type 2 diabetes is treated at first by changes to the diet, as outlined below. If this does not give enough improvement then tablets may be added, and some people also go on to insulin injections if their sugar levels remain hard to control.

2 The second aim for all diabetic people is to encourage them to be as healthy as possible in other ways. This means getting weight under control (which on its own can give a huge improvement in blood sugar levels in type 2 diabetes), avoiding smoking, monitoring and treating blood pressure, checking and treating cholesterol level, and encouraging general fitness. Getting regular exercise has all sorts of benefits, including:
   • regulating blood sugar levels
   • helping insulin to work more effectively
   • reducing weight
   • improving cholesterol and blood pressure
   • keeping the heart stronger and healthier
   • reducing stress and promoting good sleep.
3 The third aim is to keep diabetes under regular review to check that control remains good and to look out for any early signs of complications. The earlier any problems are picked up, the sooner they can be tackled, and so regular monitoring is a vital part of diabetic care.

What is a 'diabetic diet'?

In days gone by people used to believe that diabetics needed to eat a special diet, but that is not true. In fact we could all do with eating a 'diabetic diet' because it simply means a healthy diet! *The Balance of Good Health* – referred to throughout this book – contains the ideal diet for someone with diabetes because it focuses on getting the right balance of healthy foods without too much of the less healthy ingredients.

In particular, someone with diabetes should:

• eat at least three meals per day, each including starchy foods such as multigrain bread, potatoes, rice or pasta. These foods release glucose into the bloodstream more slowly than sugary foods, so that the person's insulin has a better chance of working effectively
• eat plenty of fruit, vegetables, wholegrain cereals and pulses
• go for sugar-free drinks
• limit sugary foods or foods with a high glycaemic index (*see* Chapter 12)
• reduce the fat content of the diet
• watch out for added salt and reduce salt intake
• aim to eat healthily most days of the week, even if they do not manage it every day.

Foods labelled 'for diabetics' are unnecessary and often expensive. Instead, sort out the basics of a healthy diet using *The Balance of Good Health*, and seek advice from a registered dietician to boost knowledge and confidence at the beginning. Most people who are newly diagnosed will be referred to a dietician by their family doctor as part of their initial care.

Diarrhoea

The cause of most bouts of diarrhoea is usually a viral infection, producing a sudden illness that may include vomiting, loss of appetite, abdominal gripes and watery diarrhoea. As with other viral infections, the symptoms usually drag on for several days or even up to a fortnight. In a young child, it is wise to get a medical assessment if diarrhoea persists for more than a few days, to ensure that there is no sign of dehydration and to clarify the cause of the symptoms.

There is no need to forbid solids but it is wise to be guided by the child's appetite. If not hungry then do not push food. However, it is very important to encourage plenty of fluids, but avoid drinks that are very sugary as these can worsen symptoms. Very dilute squash is suitable for the first day or two. If symptoms persist swap to oral rehydration sachets, which are available in pharmacies, and which provide the correct balance of sugar and salt to replace what has been lost. Because viral infections cause flu-like symptoms, including aching and general malaise, paracetamol will help settle these and will not worsen the diarrhoea.

Most diarrhoeal bugs are infectious and so take care with hygiene, hand washing and any close contact. Avoid sharing towels and kitchen utensils with the affected person.

Chronic diarrhoea

This is where diarrhoea has persisted for over two weeks. In a child, it is essential to seek a medical opinion, particularly if the child is unwell and losing weight.

'Toddler diarrhoea' is often found in children between the ages of one and two years. The child is fit and well but has persistently watery or runny motions that may contain undigested food. It may be caused by excessive intake of fluids, especially fruit juices or very sugary drinks, or by having too much fibre in the diet. It is not usually recommended to cut out milk or dairy products because this can lead to the child's growth tailing off. Consider doing a simple food diary to see if there are any obvious trigger foods and then discuss these findings with a dietician or family doctor to see if any dietary changes are logical.

Gastro-oesophageal reflux

This is a common condition in young babies where milk is brought back up after a feed. In very young babies small amounts are almost universal and it is called posseting. It may be worse if a baby is aggressively winded after a feed. As a baby matures, the valve at the top of the stomach becomes better at preventing reflux and the condition usually settles.

Occasionally, this mechanism is ineffective and the baby continues to bring up large amounts of each feed, which can cause breathing problems as well as failure to thrive. In this situation, the feed can be thickened with a special starch preparation which, when combined with a more upright feeding position, usually controls the problem.

If concerned about this condition, see your family doctor, taking your baby's growth chart with you, so that growth can be monitored.

Inflammatory conditions of the gut

There are two diseases, Crohn's disease and ulcerative colitis, that cause ulcera-tion of the small or large bowel, producing frequent bouts of diarrhoea, the passage of blood or mucus, weight loss and a general feeling of being unwell.

There may also be anaemia, arthritis and some skin conditions. Neither condition is common but both may sometimes start in childhood. If a child is unwell with persisting diarrhoea and weight loss, a family doctor will check whether these conditions could be present. If so, then specialist care will be arranged to plan treatment. This usually involves tablets but surgery is sometimes needed.

Phenylketonuria

This is a rare inherited disease where the body is unable to break down a particular amino acid called phenylalanine. This causes a dangerous build-up, which can lead to severe mental retardation. In the UK and many other countries all new babies are screened for the disorder during the first week of life. If a baby is affected, it is vital that they follow a highly restricted diet that contains no phenylalanine, particularly during the first eight to ten years but preferably for life, so that brain development and function are not impeded.

Phenylalanine is found in most natural proteins so the diet needs to exclude milk and dairy products, meat including chicken, eggs, beans and nuts, which all contain large amounts. Fruit and vegetables, bread and pasta contain less so can be included in measured amounts in the diet. Specialist advice is needed and early referral to a specialist will be arranged if this condition is picked up.

Pyloric stenosis

Pyloric stenosis is a condition that can happen early on in a new baby's life, during the first few months. It is due to a thickened band of the muscle around the gut that stops milk in the stomach from passing any further. As the muscular band develops, the baby begins to vomit after feeds, but then is eager to feed again soon after vomiting. The vomiting is usually impressive and projectile. Because the milk is not kept down, the baby can become undernourished and dehydrated.

The condition is commoner in male babies and the treatment is a small operation to divide the band of muscle.

Thyroid disorders

The thyroid gland is a small gland at the base of the neck, which produces a hormone called thyroxine. Thyroxine controls many things, including our rate of metabolism, body temperature, growth and development. The thyroid gland can be both overactive and underactive; it is so important to newborn babies that a heel-prick test is performed on all babies within the first week of life to check it is working properly.

If the gland is underactive this causes *hypothyroidism*, where metabolism and growth slow down. In a baby this will cause poor appetite, sleepiness, constipation and failure to thrive. In an older child it will cause slower growth, tiredness – especially after exercise – constipation, clumsiness and poor concentration and attention. A goitre may develop, which is a soft swelling at the base of the neck due to bulging of the thyroid gland.

If the gland is overactive this is called *hyperthyroidism*, where the metabolic rate is too fast. In a baby this will cause a fast heart rate, restlessness and a ravenous appetite but poor weight gain. If it develops in an older child it may cause difficulties with concentration, leading to disruptive behaviour and poor school performance.

At what age may a thyroid problem appear?

There are two phases of childhood in which thyroid problems arise: soon after birth and around the ages of eight to ten.

An underactive thyroid gland at birth (known as congenital hypothyroidism) is where the thyroid gland fails to develop properly. All new babies are screened for this condition because, if left untreated, it can lead to severe growth and development problems, including brain damage. It is treated by giving thyroxine every day for life, with monitoring every few months initially with a blood test.

An overactive thyroid gland at birth is very rare, but may sometimes happen in families that tend to have thyroid problems.

At around eight to ten years, particularly in families that are prone to thyroid problems, a child may begin to show signs of an underactive thyroid or, even less commonly, an overactive thyroid. Both conditions are usually an *autoimmune* problem, where the body's own immune system has started to think that the thyroid gland doesn't belong. The body's defences attack the gland and either stop it from working (hypothyroidism) or actually make it go into overdrive (hyperthyroidism).

Up until this time, the thyroid gland has just about kept pace, but as the normal growth spurt that comes before puberty starts, an underactive thyroid gland can no longer keep up and the child begins to slow down. A common sign is being shorter than others of the same age, because thyroxine is needed for bone growth. A simple blood test will give the answer if a child seems unusually tired and slow.

An overactive thyroid gland is fairly rare in childhood but may cause excessive growth because of the effect that thyroxine has on bones, in addition to behaviour and concentration problems.

Tooth decay

Although teeth seem incredibly hard, they are susceptible to attack in the form of both tooth decay and gum disease. This creates problems in four areas:

- the cosmetic appearance of teeth
- their ability to do their job, i.e. to chew food
- pain and discomfort from infections of the teeth and gums
- loss of teeth altogether from decay, dental abscess or from gum disease.

When affected by tooth decay (also known as dental caries), brown patches develop on the tooth's surface, which leads to collapse of the underlying part of the tooth, forming a cavity. Cavities can be treated by a dentist, using fillings of either silver-coloured amalgam or a whitish material that matches the rest of the tooth. However, if left untreated, infection can travel down the tooth and into the jaw where it can form an abscess. Once an abscess forms, the tooth usually has to be pulled out altogether unless root canal treatment is possible. Either way, the condition is painful and unpleasant, but happily is very much avoidable.

What causes tooth decay?

Tooth decay is caused by a combination of bacteria in the mouth plus sugar. Mouth bacteria produce plaque acids which dissolve minerals in the tooth's hard surface, leading to the brown patches referred to above. However, bacteria alone do not do much damage. It is only when there is a steady supply of sugar in the mouth that tooth decay really becomes a problem, as bacteria use sugar to produce the plaque acid that does the damage. The acid attack that bacteria plus sugar produces takes about 20 minutes to fade away, and each time more sugar arrives in the mouth, bacteria wake up and do more damage.

Eating lots of acidic foods causes further damage in a slightly different way, by causing dental erosion. This is where the hard enamel surface of the teeth is thinned or worn away, leaving teeth that feel sensitive to hot and cold and are at greater risk of decay.

What causes gum disease?

Gum disease is caused by plaque, which is the slimy film of bacteria that builds up on teeth. When this forms next to the gum it can cause infection and damage, making the gums sore, sensitive and likely to bleed easily. If gum disease persists, it can lead to teeth becoming loose and thus at increased risk of infection.

It is best to use a toothbrush with a small head and soft bristles, in order not to damage the gums when brushing teeth.

How may tooth decay and dental erosion be avoided?

There are three different approaches that, in combination, will greatly reduce the chance of tooth decay and dental erosion:

1 *Tooth brushing*. Teeth should be brushed twice a day using fluoride toothpaste, ensuring that impacted food is completely removed from the surface of the back teeth in particular. This routine should start as soon as babies begin to cut their teeth, using a very soft baby toothbrush, in order to help the baby get used to the process. Parents should supervise and help with every brushing in children under the age of about seven, whilst children up to around 10 years should have their tooth brushing double-checked to ensure they are doing it effectively. Fluoride toothpaste will help to refresh the mouth in addition to strengthening teeth against decay, because fluoride is an essential part of tooth enamel.

2 *Eating and drinking*. Sugar between meals causes tooth decay and so cutting this out is a great way to protect teeth. The longer the mouth is empty between meals, the better it is for teeth. Sugary foods can be eaten at mealtimes without worry, but if snacks are wanted in between meals then they should be low or preferably absent in sugar. See the section on safe snacks in the Food Frequency Framework for further ideas (page 163). Candy, sweets, chocolate and sweetened drinks should all be reserved for mealtimes in order to have least effect on teeth. If they are eaten between meals, they should be consumed as quickly as possible instead of sucked or eaten slowly, in order to cause least damage. Fizzy drinks, even low-sugar varieties, as well as fruit

juice, have a bad effect on teeth because they are acidic, which can lead to dental erosion in addition to tooth decay, and so they are best kept to a minimum and consumed at mealtimes rather than between meals.

3 *Visiting the dentist.* Regular dental check-ups are important for children as well as adults, even if teeth appear to be in good shape. The dentist will look for any early signs of tooth decay and give help and advice on good tooth brushing and general mouth hygiene. The dentist may recommend 'disclosing tablets' to teach children to clean teeth well and find out if there are areas that their toothbrush tends to miss.

Worms

Despite the 'ugh!' factor, worms are one of the commonest infestations of childhood and feature on every child's predictable trouble list along with coughs, colds, tummy ache and head lice. Whilst the majority are fairly harmless, most families prefer their 'pets' to dwell in less personal places and so careful attention to hygiene will help in breaking the cycle of reinfection. The eggs of all worms are tiny and are easily picked up in the community; becoming infested is not a sign of poor hygiene or an unhealthy lifestyle, it is just bad luck.

Threadworms are common worldwide, but other varieties such as tapeworms and roundworms may occasionally be picked up, particularly if travelling abroad.

Threadworms

These are tiny clear or whitish wriggling worms that are often noticed after passing a motion. They cause itching around the back passage, but young children will often appear to be more squirmy or fidgety than usual. Scratching down below, especially at night, causes the eggs of the threadworm to be gathered under fingernails, which can then easily be transferred back into the mouth. This causes the cycle of reinfection. The eggs are invisible and are very easy to pick up or pass on to other people, so the infection can easily spread.

Treatment involves two steps: the first is to kill off the adult threadworms with a medication such as mebendazole or piperazine, which are both available over the counter in pharmacies or via a family doctor. All the family should be treated at the same time. The second step is crucial in order to break the cycle of reinfection, because the medication will not kill any eggs that have already been laid.

• Wash hands and scrub fingernails before each meal or before picking up food.
• Wash hands and scrub fingernails after every visit to the toilet.
• Bath or shower first thing in the morning to wash away any eggs that may have been laid during the night.
• Put close-fitting underpants or pyjamas on children to reduce the chance of picking up eggs if scratching at night.

Roundworms

Despite their size of between 15 and 30 cm long, roundworms may cause no symptoms and simply be an alarming discovery after passing a motion. If the infestation is more severe they can lead to abdominal pain and blockage of the bowel, and can cause a lung infection. The treatment is the same as for thread-worms, but happily roundworms are uncommon in the UK.

Tapeworms

Tapeworms are usually more of a problem in animals, but the eggs can be transmitted to humans too. It is important to ensure that meat is properly cooked and that hands are washed after contact with animals. Tapeworm infestation is now very uncommon in the UK because of the widespread treatment of animals for tapeworm.

Height and weight charts showing normal growth

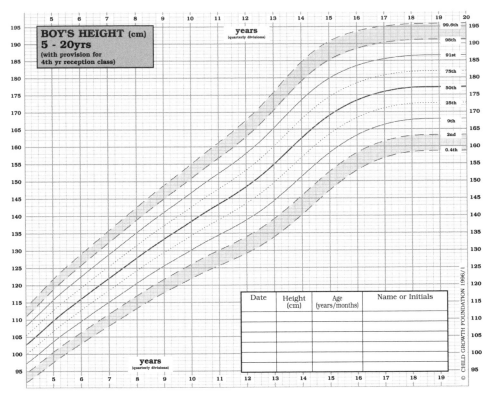

Figure A1 Boy's height (cm) from 5–20 years. Reproduced by kind permission of the Child Growth Foundation.

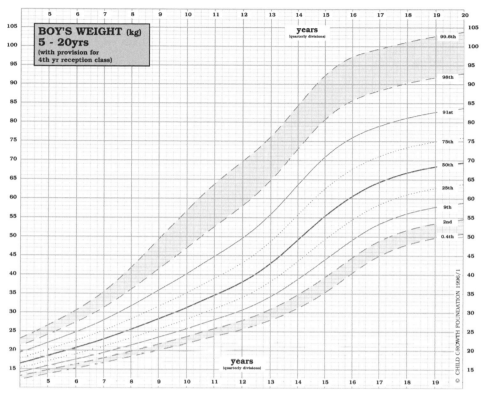

Figure A2 Boy's weight (kg) from 5–20 years. Reproduced by kind permission of the Child Growth Foundation.

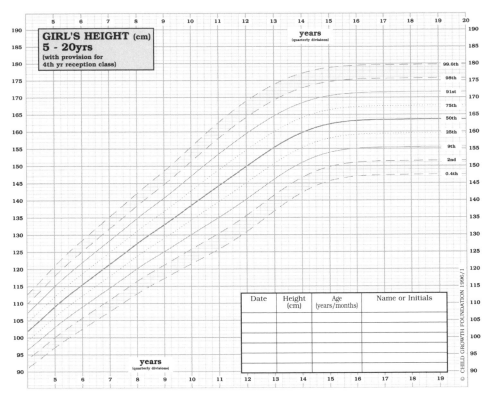

Figure A3 Girl's height (cm) from 5–20 years. Reproduced by kind permission of the Child Growth Foundation.

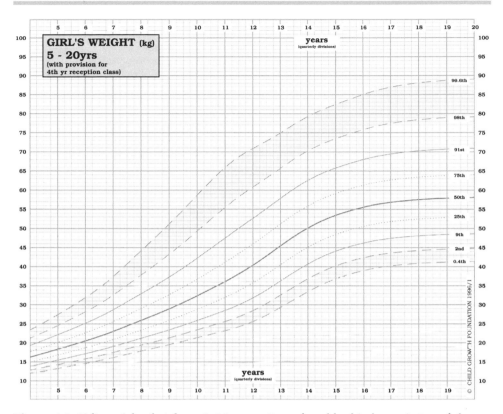

Figure A4 Girl's weight (kg) from 5–20 years. Reproduced by kind permission of the Child Growth Foundation.

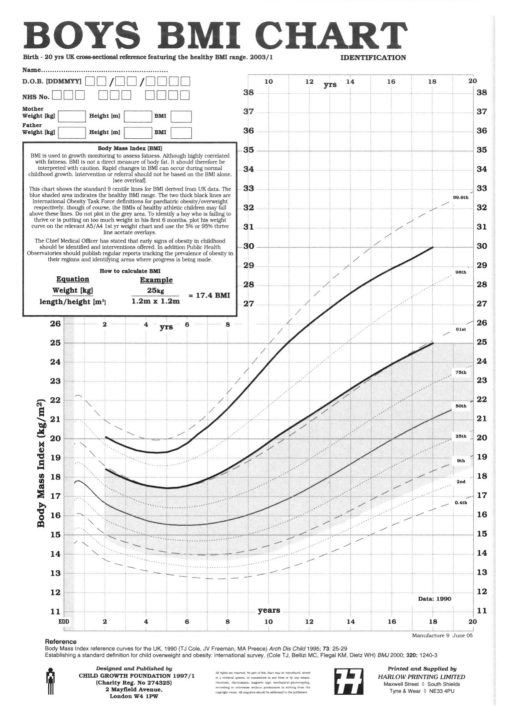

Figure A5 Boy's BMI chart up to 20 years. Reproduced by kind permission of the Child Growth Foundation.

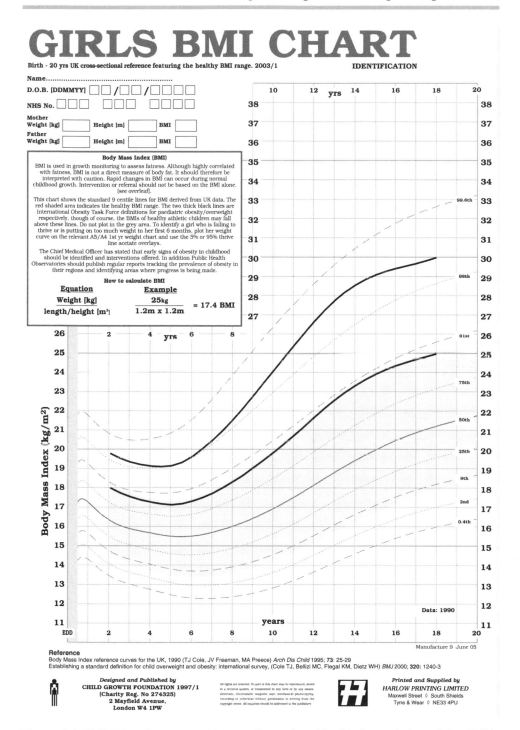

Figure A6 Girl's BMI chart up to 20 years. Reproduced by kind permission of the Child Growth Foundation.

Useful resources

Nutrition

The Dairy Council
Gives information about dairy products, including providing healthy vending in schools.
www.milk.co.uk

The Food Commission
94 White Lion Street, London N1 9PF.
Tel: 020 7837 2250
A national non-profit organisation that campaigns for the right to safe, wholesome food. The Food Commission publishes *Food Magazine*, which is the UK's leading independent food magazine covering product investigations, the latest news on diet and health, and ideas on how people can help campaign for safer, healthier food for them and their family.
www.foodcomm.org.uk

Food Standards Agency
Tel: 020 7276 8000
An independent food safety watchdog set up by an Act of Parliament in 2000 to protect the public's health and consumer interests in relation to food. Their main website is www.food.gov.uk. They also have a great site for families and young people, giving a wide range of nutritional information plus the chance to post your own email questions, at www.eatwell.gov.uk.

Health Education Trust
Tel: 01789 773915
A UK registered charity formed to boost the development of health education for young people. It campaigns on topics such as improvements in school meals and action on healthier school food and drink vending.
www.healthedtrust.com

La Leche League
For breast-feeding information and support.
Helpline: 0845 120 2918
www.laleche.org.uk

National Childbirth Trust (NCT)
Enquiry line: 0870 444 8707 (8:30 am to 5 pm, Monday to Thursday; 8:30 am to 4 pm, Fridays)
Breast-feeding line: 0870 444 8708 (8 am to 10 pm, seven days a week)
Membership hotline: 0870 990 8040 to join the NCT using a credit or debit card
www.nctpregnancyandbabycare.com/nct-online

The Parent's Jury
Tel: 020 7837 2250
An independent jury of over 1300 parents, co-ordinated by The Food Commission, who seek to improve the quality of children's food and drinks in the UK. They have been instrumental in promoting healthy change with campaigns such as Chuck Snacks off the Checkout.
www.parentsjury.org.uk

Organic food and farming

Information about organic food and farming is available through the following:

Henry Doubleday Foundation
www.hdra.org.uk

Fish stocks and safe fishing practices
Further information about sustainable fishing and how consumers can help can be found at www.fishonline.org.

The Soil Association
www.soilassociation.org

The Vegan Society
Donald Watson House, 7 Battle Road, St Leonards-on-Sea, East Sussex TN37 7AA
Tel: 01424 427393
www.vegansociety.com

The Vegetarian Society
Parkdale, Dunham Road, Altrincham, Cheshire WA14 4QG
Tel: 0161 925 2000; Fax: 0161 926 9182
www.vegsoc.org

Recommended cookbooks

- *Annabel Karmel's Favourite Family Recipes.* Ebury Press. An ideal guide to easy family meals.

- *Ainsley Harriott's All New Meals in Minutes.* Dorling Kindersley. Quick meals that will go down well with all the family.

- *Sophie Grigson's Country Kitchen.* Headline. Fabulous ideas for incorporating fruit and vegetables into meals throughout the year.

- Nigel Slater. *Real Fast Food.* Penguin. A timeless guide to fast easy nutrition for busy families.

- *Delia Smith's Complete Cookery Course.* BBC Books. The ultimate reference book for anyone wanting to cook fail-safe traditional meals that the whole family will appreciate.

Health

Asthma UK
Advice line: 08457 01 02 03 (9 am to 5 pm, Monday to Friday)
In addition to their telephone advice line, they have an email information service through the website, plus a very useful 'kidszone' page.
www.asthma.org.uk

The British Heart Foundation
Tel: 0870 600 6566
This charity has many initiatives to boost health for adults and children, including funding research and promoting education. For further information, including their useful 'Get Kids on the Go' leaflet, go to the website www.bhf.org.uk/youngpeople, which has lots of activity and nutritional information too.

Coeliac UK
PO Box 220, High Wycombe, Bucks HP11 2HY.
Helpline: 0870 444 8804
Gives comprehensive information on the diagnosis of coeliac disease and ways to manage a gluten-free diet.
www.coeliac.co.uk

Cystic Fibrosis Trust
11 London Road, Bromley, Kent BR1 1BY
General helpline: 0845 859 1000
This national organisation works to fund research into a cure and to ensure appropriate clinical care and support for people with cystic fibrosis.
www.cftrust.org.uk

Diabetes UK
Macleod House, 10 Parkway, London NW1 7AA
Tel: 020 7424 1000; Email: info@diabetes.org.uk
Supports people with diabetes, funds research and campaigns to improve the lives of people with the condition.
www.diabetes.org.uk

Health Education Authority – Wired for Health
This is a series of websites run on behalf of the Department of Health and the Department for Education and Skills. There are four sites for young people, covering a range of health topics for different age groups ranging from 5 to 16.
www.wiredforhealth.gov.uk

Health For All Children – online growth charts
This is an ideal site for plotting a child's height and weight and calculating body mass index (BMI). Go to www.healthforallchildren.co.uk and choose the parent's page.

Institute of Child Health and Great Ormond Street Family Resource Centre
Institute of Child Health, 30 Guildford Street, London WC1N 1EH
Tel: 020 7242 9789
Great Ormond Street Family Resource Centre, Great Ormond Street, London WC1N 3JH
Tel: 020 7405 9200

The combined website of these two organisations gives comprehensive information on a huge range of illnesses in its Health A to Z, plus many other issues such as what to expect if a trip to hospital is needed.
www.childrenfirst.nhs.uk or www.ich.ucl.ac.uk

NHS Direct
Tel: 0845 4647
This freephone service is staffed by nurses to give immediate information and guidelines on health and illness. There is also a comprehensive website giving health and illness advice at www.nhsdirect.nhs.uk.

Smoking cessation advice services

ASH – Action on Smoking and Health UK
In addition to English-speaking services there are a number of support lines in foreign languages. Details are on the website.
www.ash.org.uk

NHS Pregnancy Smoking Helpline
Tel: 0800 169 9 169 (12 noon to 9 pm, seven days a week. Answerphone out of hours)

NHS Smoking Helpline
Tel: 0800 169 0 169 (7 am to 11 pm, seven days a week)

Quitline
Tel: 0800 002 200
www.quit.org.uk

Activity and exercise

Disability Sport England
This organisation gives information on getting involved in sports for disabled people, charity information and details on sponsorship. It also lists a calendar of Disability Sport England events.
www.disabilitysport.org.uk/

Hyperactive Children's Support Group
71 Whyke Lane, Chichester, West Sussex PO19 7PD
Tel: 01243 551313; Email: hyperactive@hacsg.org.uk
This charity organisation provides support for attention deficit hyperactivity disorder (ADHD)/hyperactive children and their families, encouraging a dietary approach to the problem of hyperactivity.
www.hacsg.org.uk

Sport England
This organisation takes the strategic lead for sport in England, creating opportunities for people to start, stay and succeed in sport. Its website gives details of clubs and facilities in local areas.
http://www.sportengland.org

Sports Coach UK
For information on coaching at every level in the UK.
www.sportscoachuk.org

Sustrans – cycle routes
Information service: 0845 113 0065; E-mail: info@sustrans.org.uk for details.
This charity works on practical projects to encourage people to walk, cycle and use public transport and gives ideas on cycle routes in local areas.
www.sustrans.org.uk

Toy library
There are toy libraries up and down the country, offering good quality toys on loan either free or for a nominal charge. Search on the internet under 'toy library' plus the name of your nearest town, or try a local book library for more information.

Travel to school
Further information on setting up a walking bus and other active ways to get to school can be found on these websites.
www.walkingbus.com and www. saferroutestoschool.co.uk

Safety information for children's play

The Children's Play Council
Promotes play initiatives and campaigns for safe and accessible play areas for children.
http://www.ncb.org.uk/cpc and www.playday.org.uk

Royal Society for the Prevention of Accidents
Provides information relating to safe play.
www.rospa.co.uk/playsafety

Emotional health

ChildLine
Helpline: 0800 1111
ChildLine is the UK's free, 24-hour helpline for children in distress or danger. Trained volunteer counsellors comfort, advise and protect children and young people who may feel they have nowhere else to turn.
www.childline.org.uk

Media Smart
A website that aims to help six to 11 year-olds develop the skills they need to interpret, understand and think critically about the media and advertising. Leaflets and practical tips are available online at
www.mediasmart.org.uk/parents.

Parentline Plus
Freephone helpline: 0808 800 2222 (available 24 hours a day)
This national charity works for and with parents to give guidance on a wealth of topics from bullying, divorce and discipline through to drugs and talking about

relationships. An email reply service is available through the website www. parentlineplus.org.uk.

Samaritans

Tel: 08457 909090; Email Jo@samaritans.org

Confidential emotional support is available 24 hours a day by telephone, letter, e-mail and minicom, if people are experiencing feelings of distress or despair, including those which may lead to suicide. Some local offices also provide face-to-face contact.

Look in the *Yellow Pages* for a local phone number as they have over 200 support offices.

www.samaritans.org.uk

Young Minds

Tel: 0800 018 2138

This national charity is committed to improving the mental health of all children and young people. They provide leaflets and booklets plus a parents' information service. The website has pages for young people and for parents, as well as information for professionals involved in helping young people.

www. youngminds.org.uk

Index

Page numbers in *italics* refer to tables or figures.

WITHDRAWN
FROM STOCK
QMUL LIBRARY